Contents

Barefoot/Macrobiotic Shiatsu 1
Fundamentals of Health 7
Macrobiotics 8
Life-style Guidelines 11
Cause of Illness 12
Health 15
Chinese Medical Foundations 16
Source of Blood 24
Sources of Energy (Qi) 25
Energy Flow Within The Body 26
Spiral of Creation 26
Face Diagnosis 27
Internal Organs, Emotions, and Facial Diagnosis 28
Back and Front Points 29
Major Energy Centers (Chakras) 30
Shiatsu Techniques 31
Abdominal Organs 32
Barefoot/Macrobiotic Shiatsu Treatment 33
Self-Shiatsu Treatment (Do-In) 40
Meridians 42
    Lung 42
    Large Intestine 47
    Spleen 49
    Stomach 52
    Heart 55
    Small Intestine 58
    Kidney 60
    Bladder 64
    Liver 66
    Gall Bladder 70
    Heart Governor 73
    Tripe Heater (Sanjiao) 75
    Governing Vessel 78
    Conception Vessel 80
Summary of Meridian Pathology 82
Circulating Direction of the Meridians 83
Natural Home Remedies 84
Acupoint Names 100
About the Authors 107

Copyright © 2006 Shizuko Yamamoto & Patrick McCarty
All Rights Reserved

The medical and heath procedures in this book are based on training, personal experiences, and research of the author. Because each person and situation is unique, the editor and the publisher urge the reader to check with a qualified health professional before using any procedure where there is any question as to its appropriateness.

The publisher does not advocate the use of any particular diet or exercise program but believes the information presented in this book should be available to the public.

Because there is always some risk involved, the author and publisher are not responsible for any adverse effects or consequences resulting from the use of any of the suggestions, preparations, or procedures in this book. Please do not use the book if you are unwilling to assume the risk. Feel free to consult a physician or other qualified health professional. It is a sign of wisdom, not cowardice, to seek a second or third opinion.

Copyright © 2006 by Shizuko Yamamoto & Patrick McCarty

All rights reserved. No part of this publication may be reproduced, stored in a retrieval system, or transmitted, in any form or by any means, electronic, mechanical, photocopying, recording or otherwise, without the prior written consent of the copyright owner.

Printed in the United States of America
Intl. Macrobiotic Shiatsu Society   www.imss.macrobiotic.net

Macrobiotic Shiatsu

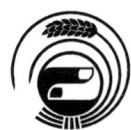

Macrobiotic/Barefoot Shiatsu is an educational and transformational healing technique. This program is designed to give essential skills to practitioners for both professional and family-style treatment. Macrobiotic Shiatsu includes techniques and exercises which stimulate the skeletal, nervous and circulatory systems, and all the major internal organs, to focus on developing refined strategies for self-correction and improved, vibrant health. Linking mind and body awareness encourages the ability to perceive obvious and subtle body movements and rhythms, awareness of one's tension, and respiratory patterns. The goal is to develop lifetime skills to promote health, happiness, and wholeness.

THEORY OF SHIATSU & PREVENTIVE HEALTH CARE

When someone is hurting either physically or emotionally our human instinct is to reach out and comfort that person. This intuitive response is the foundation of shiatsu — instinct comes first, techniques follow. Given the proper attitude of caring, technique will always naturally develop.

In Japanese the word *shi* means finger and *atsu* means pressure. Shiatsu, also called acupressure, is an Asian healing method in which specific points on the surface of the body are pressed.

Energy (*Qi* or *Ki*) tends to stagnate in specific points along the meridian (pathway of energy) called acupoints. There are hundreds of acupoints on the human body. When energy is blocked in an acupoint, it becomes sensitive to pressure. In shiatsu the acupoints are pressed to stimulate the movement of stagnated energy as well as to diagnose the presence of disease.

Symptoms of illness are protective mechanisms. If we listen and heed the warning then further development is avoided.

Shiatsu never cures the patient. It is the patient who heals himself. The practitioner is the stimulus to aid the patient in assuming a proper direction. The practitioner serves as a mirror for the patient, allowing the patient the opportunity to self-reflect on the true cause of his or her condition. Our approach is educational.

Shiatsu creates a deep feeling of well-being, vitality, and relaxation, and is an effective tool in preventing disease. Shiatsu can be a pleasurable experience. It encourages communication between family members, couples, and friends. It requires no special equipment, oil, or the removal of clothes. It can be done anywhere, at anytime.

ORIGIN OF SHIATSU

Since the beginning of time people have used various styles of touch to try to soothe and heal family and friends. While scholars feel that massage originated in China it is certain that each country throughout the world had developed and passed down their methods for treating the body with the hands. Ancient writings of Egypt, Persia, Greece, Rome, and Asian countries mention the positive effects from the use of massage.

We instinctively rub, press, pat, or in some way touch when we ache, feel pain, or just don't feel right. Intuitively we are applying self-treatment to try to create a more balanced state. Everyone is qualified to help themselves and with a little effort, are able to help others too. The simple understanding that humans are equipped to heal themselves, and that we can also help others, is the underlying foundation of shiatsu. If we live according to natural laws we really shouldn't have many troubles. Unfortunately we don't consistently live that way and humankind has had to devise ways to deal with the suffering that we experience. Ultimately to regain wholeness we must change our way of living. There are many tools that we can use in this process. Shiatsu is one of them.

The origin of the Japanese word "shiatsu" is not certain. Over the centuries, information that makes up the shiatsu techniques was gathered through trial and error. The healing techniques that are fundamental to shiatsu probably originated in ancient China, and later came to Japan. Shiatsu is a synthesis of Judo principles, Do-In (self massage), and ancient massage.

In 1955, the Japanese parliament adopted a bill on revised Amma treatment (ancient Asian massage). Thus, for the first time in Japan, shiatsu was given official endorsement.

Neither a thorough physical checkup by a doctor of Western medicine, nor a complete laboratory analysis, can adequately diagnose and cure symptoms caused by nervous and mental disorders and the imbalance of the autonomic nervous system. Shiatsu is a system that has developed from centuries of experience, and has proven effective in curing many symptoms. Among these symptoms are headaches, dizziness, ringing in the ears, eyestrain, general fatigue, stiff neck and shoulders, lower backache, constipation, numbness of limbs, chills, flushes, insomnia, and lack of appetite. Shiatsu and related techniques have also proven effective for curing chronic and painful conditions such as high blood pressure, rheumatism, and general neuralgia.

THE DEVELOPMENT OF MACROBIOTIC SHIATSU

Shiatsu practitioners have long been considered authorities on treating minor diseases in Japan. In general, the Japanese public favors shiatsu treatment and, for many years, these practitioners have played a major role in health maintenance.

The practice of eating large amounts of animal food has created bodies that are very tight and rigid. To effectively deal with this hard, stiff situation an appropriate shiatsu technique naturally evolved. The Macrobiotic Shiatsu style developed as a response to the western condition. It is a technique that deals with the common problems that many Westerners have. The aim of treatment is to create balance within the individual. We are always attentive to the needs of the receiver.

The most important underlying principle of macrobiotic shiatsu is that everyone has the power to heal themselves. This power comes as standard equipment with each human being. In a very practical way every shiatsu session is in reality a life-style education session.

This style of shiatsu developed to include both the skills that had been learned from formal training in Japan that primarily used the fingers and hands, and an intuitive foot technique. Additionally, beyond the formal training and martial arts exposure, intuition and common sense blend into the technique to make it what it is today. Its principal beauty is that it has a large sense of caring for others, of course, in a very practical way.

PRINCIPLES OF MACROBIOTIC SHIATSU

1. Health is the natural condition of human beings.
2. Illness and unhappiness are unnatural conditions.
3. Health or sickness is not an accident or something without explanation.
4. Sickness arises from how we live because of our own actions and thoughts.
5. Food is one of the more important factors in determining health or sickness.
6. We should eat foods that grow in our environment.
7. The strong will naturally help the weak.
8. People will naturally help themselves.
9. Through interaction with others, you naturally develop beyond your limitations of Body, Mind, and Spirit.

10. Purpose of treatment is to stimulate people to go beyond their previous limitations.

PREVENTIVE MEDICINE

Preventive Medicine should involve two basic approaches. The patient must cultivate proper personal habits of health and hygiene, and the practitioner must detect illnesses to which the patient is prone and give treatment and life-style suggestions before disease manifests. The first approach includes such measures as proper diet, plenty of exercise, proper breathing, regulated sex life, and other daily preventive routines. We call these the fundamentals of health. Changes in season and weather must be met by appropriate adjustments in diet and other routines so that the optimum relative balance of energies within and outside the body is maintained. This personal daily approach to preventive care is especially effective in preventing chronic and degenerative diseases from developing. It also raises one's general level of health, vitality, and resistance to infectious diseases.

The second part of the preventive approach depends on the skills of the shiatsu practitioner. The various forms of diagnosis used in Macrobiotic Shiatsu can detect existing troubles and/or give valuable information about impending troubles that may develop if not attended to. Observation of a patient's skin color, tongue, texture of hair, tone of voice, abdominal condition, bowel and urinary habits, and many other telltale signs give an accurate picture of where the patient has been and perhaps more importantly, where he or she is going. If the conditions that make the body vulnerable are corrected early enough, disease is prevented. It is the combined efforts of the skilled practitioner and the diligence of the patient that determines if prevention will be successful.

The other major addition that Macrobiotic Shiatsu includes is total treatment. The arsenal of tools used is not limited to acupressure, massage, or body work. It is from understanding the underlying reasons for ill health, such as the patient's breathing patterns, emotional changes, dietary preferences, and so on, that we get our direction concerning what must be adjusted in the patient's life-style. Besides treating the patient with shiatsu, we must look into the fundamentals of health and make appropriate adjustments in these areas also. Therefore a patient's shortsightedness in his or her life outlook is often-times pointed out. When inappropriate breathing patterns are noted, appropriate exercises are suggested. Physical movement such as yoga and walking, dietary recommendations, pointers on relationships, sex, and sleeping patterns are some of the counseling given to the receiver of Macrobiotic Shiatsu. Any area that is weak is fortified with suggestion and homework. All aspects of an individual's life are treated. This is what we mean by total treatment. This total approach affects the cause of disease by rectifying the energy imbalances and tonifying the weak organs that permit disease to develop. It also adjusts the living patterns that promote the disease in the first place.

The concepts of change, preventive care, and total treatment, traditional in Asian medicine, are recognized as integral and important elements in Macrobiotic Shiatsu.

THE MACROBIOTIC STYLE

This Macrobiotic style of shiatsu coordinates the breathing of the giver and the receiver as an important part of the treatment. Breathing together creates a lot of energy that is used in the correcting process. A vigorous style, which includes not only pressing with the hands and thumbs but the use of the giver's whole body, helps to loosen up the stiffness that so many people have. Stretching is also an important element of this style. In the diagnosis segment of a shiatsu session the senses of touch, vision and smell plus the intuitive sense are used. By understanding the imbalances that are present, accurate way of life recommendations can be made.

This holistic style of treatment teaches the importance of diet, breathing, and corrective exercise to be included with shiatsu treatment. In short, it has always included life-style adjustments. These methods are used because they are effective.

In sharing shiatsu, you are participating in the healing arts at a high level. The act of treating someone provides a powerful means of personal growth for the practitioner in a similar way that the practice of the martial arts allows an adept's spiritual nature to develop. The essence of shiatsu is Love, which is infinitely available. It's no wonder that after a shiatsu session both giver and receiver are smiling.

FUNDAMENTALS OF HEALTH

1. Consciousness
2. Breathing
3. Movement
4. Diet
5. Elimination
6. Relationships and Sex
7. Sleep

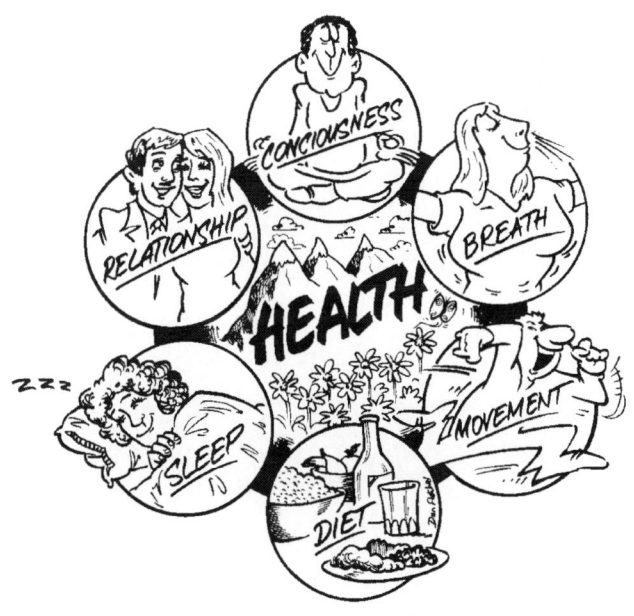

Macrobiotics

Macrobiotics is a way of eating and living that has been practiced for thousands of years by many people around the world. It stems from an intuitive understanding of the orderliness of nature. Modern macrobiotic philosophy focuses on offering a way of living that closes the widening gap between humans and the natural world. Macrobiotic theory suggests that sickness and unhappiness are nature's way of urging us to adopt a proper diet and way of life, and that these troubles are unnecessary when we live in harmony with our environment. The macrobiotic diet is based on whole grains and traditional foods in harmony with the seasons.

— Michio Kushi

General Principles of Eating

- Increase complex carbohydrates (such as whole grains & vegetables)
- Eliminate refined carbohydrates and processed sugar
- Reduce fat (especially fat from animal sources)
- Reduce cholesterol-rich foods (beef, chicken, cheese, etc.)
- Eliminate refined salt (use good quality sea salt)
- Avoid junk food
- Don't overeat and be sure to chew well

Create Variety In Your Cooking

Select organic foods within the following categories: whole grains, soup, seasonal vegetables, beans, sea vegetables, condiments, pickles, beverages, and occasionally fish, fruit, nuts, and seeds.

Use different cooking methods such as:

Most Frequently-Pressure Cooking, Steaming, Stewing, Water Sautéing, Boiling, Blanching, Marinating, Pressed Salad, Pickling.

Less Frequently-Oil Sautéing, Stir Frying, Deep Frying, Tempura, Baking, Raw salad, Dry roast, Barbecue.

Cut vegetables in different ways.

Vary amount of water used.

Vary kinds of seasonings and condiments.

Vary cooking time-do not overcook or pressure cook vegetables.

Adjust cooking to seasonal changes.

Macrobiotic Dietary Recommendations

1. **WHOLE CEREAL GRAINS**. Between 40-60% of the volume of every meal should include cooked whole cereal grains prepared in a variety of ways. Whole cereal grains include brown rice, barley, millet, oats, corn, rye, wheat, and buckwheat. It is best that only a small portion of this amount be taken as flour products in the forms of noodles, unyeasted whole grain breads, and other partially processed products, because flour products tend to be more difficult to digest and create excess mucus more easily than the whole grains.

2. **SOUPS**. Approximately 5% of your daily food intake should include miso, tamari (shoyu) broth, or vegetable soup (one or two bowls). The flavor should not be overly salty.

3. **VEGETABLES**. A wide variety of vegetables should be used daily. Approximately 25-35% of each meal should be used.

4. **BEANS**. Approximately 10-15% of your daily diet should include cooked beans and bean products such as tempeh, tofu, and natto.

5. **SEA VEGETABLES**. High in necessary minerals approximately 5% of your daily diet should include sea vegetables such as nori, hijiki, wakame, kombu, arame, & dulse.

6. **SUPPLEMENTAL FOODS**. A small portion of a variety of other foods such as fish, fruit, nuts, and seeds should be included in the diet.

7. **BEVERAGES**. Recommended daily beverages include roasted twig tea (kukicha), roasted brown rice tea, roasted barley tea, cereal grain coffee, and other traditional teas that do not have strong aromatic properties and stimulating effects can be used.

8. **FOODS TO AVOID**. Meat, eggs, animal fat, poultry, sugar, and dairy products including butter, yogurt, ice cream, cheese, and milk. All artificially colored, preserved, sprayed, or chemically treated foods are also best avoided.

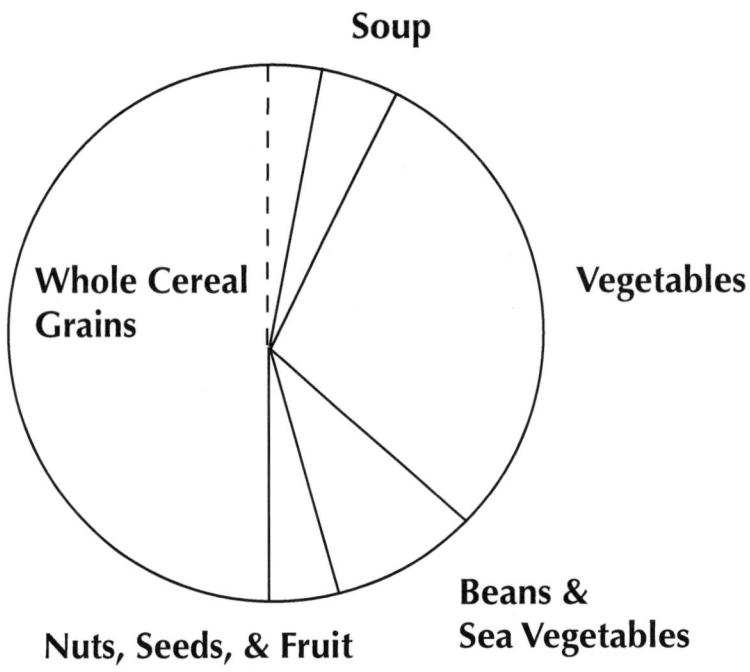

Life-style Guidelines

- Be happy and don't worry.

- Eat when you are hungry, drink when you are thirsty.

- Eat only to 80% capacity of your appetite.

- Chew every mouthful until it becomes liquid.

- Avoid eating 3 hours before going to bed.

- Go to bed before midnight.

- Scrub and massage your body everyday with a damp towel until the skin becomes pink.

- Keep your house and personal belongings clean and orderly.

- Wear natural fiber clothing such as cotton, linen, silk, and wool.

- Spend time outside everyday and exercise regularly.

- It is advised to use gas or wood stoves for cooking, rather than electric or microwave cooking.

- Use earthenware, cast iron, or stainless steel cookware rather than aluminum or teflon coated pots.

- Avoid using chemically produced cosmetics or toothpaste.

Cause of Illness

When the parts and energies in the body are in harmonious balance, there is health. When this balance is disturbed, there is illness. Illness is the absence of health. Illness occurs when there is a separation or cutting off of vital life-force. There are two causes that separate humankind from our natural state of health: **External Causes and Internal Causes**.

The activities of the Blood, Organs, Qi, Meridians, Body Fluids, Essence and Spirit are considered Normal Qi. The course of disease is seen as a struggle between the Normal Qi and the disease causing elements. It is this struggle which produces symptoms.

SIX EXTERNAL CAUSES OF ILLNESS (Exogenous Factors)

WIND

Diseases caused by Wind arise suddenly and change quickly. They may be accompanied by symptoms such as spasm, vertigo, itching, or a pain which often changes location. Wind diseases from external sources usually affect the skin, head, throat, and lungs first (e.g. colds and flu). Wind is the excess which carries other excesses into the body.

Internally, when the Liver Yang is hyperactive, dizziness, convulsions, etc. occur, sometimes accompanied with high fevers. Both are call Interior Wind.

COLD

The principle symptom of this Excess is that the body, or part of the body, feels cold. Cold causes things to congeal; in the body this causes pain. Pain is caused by obstruction in the flow of Qi or Blood. Cold causes things to contract; in the meridians this causes cramps and spasms. When Cold diseases are present, the body excretions such as mucus, phlegm, urine, stool, etc. are white or clear and watery.

When the Yang Qi is weak, symptoms similar to those caused by Cold appear.

HEAT

The main symptoms of this Excess is that the body, or part of the body, feels hot. Heat easily injures body fluids. Therefore the patient is thirsty and the tongue and stool can become dry. Heat can cause the Blood to travel outside the meridians leading to hemorrhage or rashes. Body excretions are usually dark or yellow, sticky and/or foul smelling. Often times disease caused by one of the other excesses transforms into Heat within the body. Heat is sometimes called Fire.

SUMMER HEAT

The primary characteristic of Summer Heat is fever with pronounced sweating. Onset occurs only in summer and is often due to prolonged exposure to sun on hot days, or staying in a hot room with poor ventilation. Additionally, thirst, shortness of breath, lassitude, and concentrated urine can occur. This injures the Yin and the Qi. Damp can accompany Summer Heat (like summer storms) and leads to dizziness, a heavy sensation in the head, suffocating feel in the chest, nausea, poor appetite, diarrhea, and general sluggishness.

DAMPNESS

This Excess often appears during damp weather or when a person comes in contact with moisture for a prolonged period of time. Dampness is sluggish and stagnating. Damp diseases take a long time to cure. When dampness is on the external parts of the body, the patient feels pent-up, limbs feel heavy, and the head swollen. When Dampness invades the meridians and joints, movement is difficult, numbness may appear, and if there is pain, it is fixed in one place. The entire body or a part is affected by swelling or edema. Dampness tends to attack the Spleen. When the Spleen's transforming and transporting functions are weak, Interior Dampness may occur.

DRYNESS

Dryness attacks the fluids in the body resulting in dry skin, chapped lips, hacking cough, constipation and so forth. When the body's Yin substances are seriously depleted such as in the late states of a long bout with fever, similar symptoms appear.

SEVEN INTERNAL CAUSES OF ILLNESS (Endogenous Factors)

The seven emotions are reflections of man's mental state. They are natural and should not cause disease under normal conditions. However, if the emotions are very intense and persistent or the individual is hypersensitive, they may lead to disease.

Diseases caused by the seven emotional factors often show dysfunction of **Zang-Fu** organs and disturbance in circulation of Qi and Blood. Different emotional changes selectively injure different Organs.

SEVEN EMOTIONS	ZANG ORGANS AFFECTED
Excitability / Excess Joy	Heart
Anger	Liver
Worry	Spleen
Grief	Lung
Sadness / Melancholy	Lung
Fear	Kidney
Terror	Heart

Disorders are seen mainly in the Heart, Liver, and Spleen.

Excessive joy or fear and terror may cause mental restlessness and give rise to palpitation, insomnia, irritability, anxiety, and even mental disorders.

Excessive anger may cause dysfunction of the liver promoting pain and distension in the rib and middle region of the body, irregular menstruation, and depression.

Excessive grief, melancholy, and worry may affect the Spleen and Stomach to cause anorexia and abdominal fullness and distension after meals.

Health

KI KETSU DO

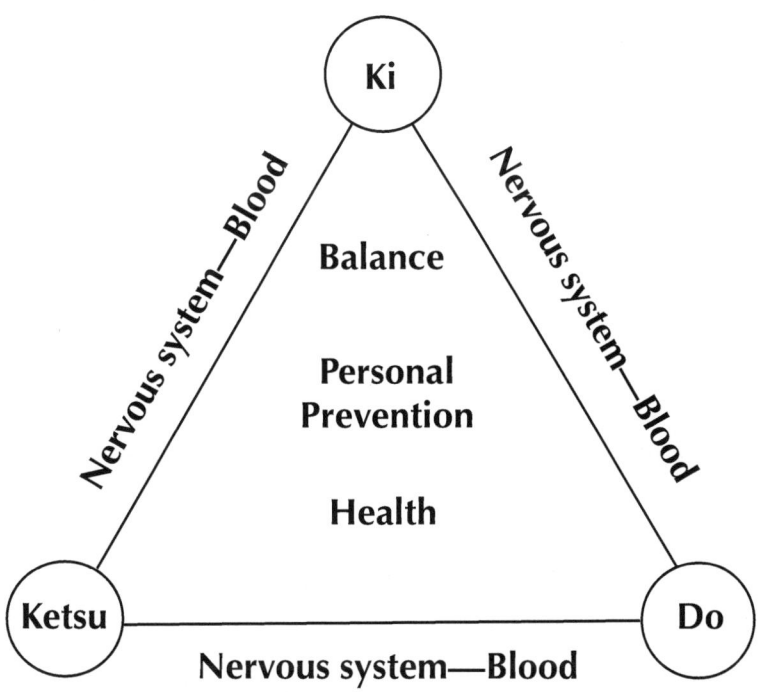

Health is more than merely being without sickness or symptoms. It is a dynamic state in which the mental, physical, and spiritual vibrations harmonize. The key to health is prevention. In Japan there is a saying: "Ki ketsu ei ei." This is the formula for good health. *Ki* is life force, *ketsu* is good quality blood, and *ei ei* is proper nourishment. Our daily food, being proper human nourishment, will make good quality blood, Ki flows in a body with good quality blood.

Macrobiotic Shiatsu Workbook

Chinese Medical Foundations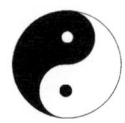

Shiatsu, as well as other natural healing modalities such as acupuncture and herbalogy perform certain functions in Traditional Chinese Medicine. They regulate the flow of Qi through the meridians and Organs, remove blockages, strengthen the body's protective energy (Qi) and lessen the noxious effect of excesses.

FUNDAMENTAL PRINCIPLES

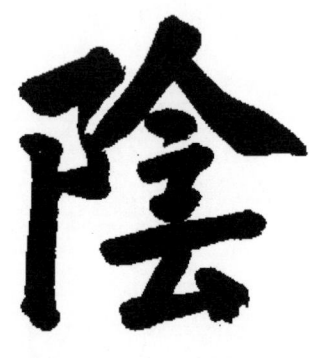 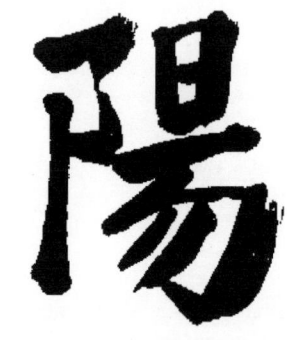

YIN	YANG
negative	positive
passive	active
female	male
receptive	creative
dark	light
night	day
cold	heat
soft	hard
wet	dry
winter	summer
shadow	sun

1. **Yin and Yang** (symbolized in the *Taiji* or "Great Polarity")

2. **Five Elements** (also known as Phases or Transformations)

   Wood is associated with active functions of growth or increase.

   Tree-like upward energy. Morning, Spring, Windy, Waxing moon.

   Fire represents functions are that are active and nearing a maximal state.

   Fire-like active energy. Noon, Summer, Hot, Full moon.

   Metal symbolizes functions that are consolidating or solidifying.

   Metal-like gathering energy. Evening, Autumn, Dry, Waning moon.

   Water represents those functions that are in a state of floating or less structured.

   Water-like floating energy. Night, Winter, Cold, New moon.

   Earth designates balance or neutrality.

   Soil-like downward energy. Afternoon, Late summer, Humid, Half moon.

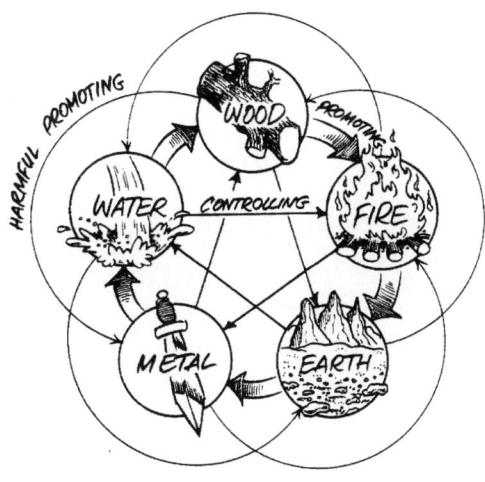

Correspondences Associated with the Five Transformations

5 Phases	Solid	Hollow	Senses	Tissues	Seasons	Environment	Color	Taste	Direction
Wood	Liver	Gall bladder	Eyes	Tendons	Spring	Wind	Green	Sour	East
Fire	Heart	Small Intestine	Tongue	Vessels	Summer	Heat	Red	Bitter	South
Earth	Spleen	Stomach	Mouth	Muscles	Late summer	Damp	Yellow	Sweet	Middle
Metal	Lung	Large Intestine	Nose	Skin/Hair	Autumn	Dryness	White	Pungent	West
Water	Kidney	Bladder	Ear	Bone	Winter	Cold	Black	Salty	North

FUNDAMENTAL PROPERTIES

3. Life Force (*Qi* or *Ki*)

Qi is an untranslatable word in the Chinese medical lexicon. It signifies a tendency, a movement, something on the order of energy. There are two main aspects of Qi. Qi is thought of as matter or substance without form. It is also thought of as the functional, active aspect of the body. While substance and function are different, they are closely related and cannot be separated.

Qi flows through the entire body and is the basis for all movement and action. Qi has different names depending on its distribution, source, and function.

Source (Yuan) Qi: the energy formed from the Essence of the Kidneys inherited from parents and ancestors. Non-renewalable. It is related to reproductive function.

Acquired Qi: from Clean/Useful (Qing) Qi & Nutrient (Ying) Qi combining.

Organ Qi: the physiological activity and functions of each Organ.

Meridian Qi: the transportive and moving functions of the meridians/channels.

Nutrient (Ying) Qi: the Qi that comes from food and drink and moves with the Blood. Its main functions are transforming and creating Blood, moving with the Blood, and helping the Blood to nourish the tissues of the body.

Protective / Defensive (Wei) Qi: the Qi that travels outside the Meridians and Organs. It comes from food. It warms the Organs, travels between the sinews and the flesh to regulate the opening and closing of the pores (thereby providing for the body's defense against external diseases), and protects and moistens the skin and hair.

Essential (Zong) Qi: the Qi that collects in the chest, with its center at point CV 17. It travels up to the throat and down into the abdomen. This Qi underlies breathing and speaking, regulates the Heart beat, and is important in strengthening the body when cultivated through meditation.

4. Meridians (Channels)

Between the third and second century B.C. the channel system was developed and described in the "Inner Classic". Frequently, when disease is present in the body, certain sites on the body's surface become spontaneously tender and painful to the touch. A patient's disease could be diagnosed by observing and probing with the fingers along the course of these areas of tenderness or pain. They are the three dimensional passageways through which Qi flows at different levels of the body. It was also theorized that these channels are connections between the surface of the body and the internal organs, sense organs, and between one area of the body and another.

The functions of the meridians are to circulate Qi and Blood, warm and nourish the tissues, and to link the whole body so as to keep the internal organs, limbs, skin, muscles, tendons, and bones intact in structure and to make the body function as a whole.

The meridian transportation system brings Qi (life force) from the surface of the body to deep into the interior and from the depths back to the surface of the body, accomplishing the job of warming and nourishing. At the same time, the meridians are responsible for the occurrence and transmission of disease. When the function of the meridian is impaired, the organism is open to attack from outside disease causing forces. Once these forces enter the body they are transmitted deep into the interior through the meridians. When external disease factors enter and block the channels, superficial symptoms appear such as chills, fever, and headache. When these forces drive deeper into the body through the meridians, organs and systems begin to decline. This is how the external disease factors influence the internal organs. Each of the meridians flow in a definite part of the body and each of the twelve regular channels connects with a different internal organ. Tenderness or other abnormal reactions along the areas the meridians pass through or at certain acupoints also aids correct diagnosis. Pain on the upper back below the shoulders indicates trouble in the lung, hot flashes suggest a disorder in the liver, and so forth. There are 14 main meridians. Twelve regular meridians and one each mid-line both front and back.

5. Acupoints (*Tsubo* or *Shuwei*)

There are special locations found along each meridian. We call these places acupoints (*tsubo* in Japanese, *shuwei* in Chinese). These points cover the entire body and extend their influence to the internal organs. Acupoints are not actually points. They are more like a hole or volcano. They are the entry and exit places for the body's energy as well as natural forces of health and illness. It is at these locations that the body's energy can easily become sluggish and stagnant. Many acupoints occur in places that are vulnerable and slightly weak. The bends of the wrists, elbows, and knees, the depressions of the muscles, and places where nerves emerge from muscles are common sites. In these spots any internal disturbance produces powerful reflex actions. The effects can be seen while the acupoints themselves are invisible. Trouble along the meridians at the acupoints is sensed as pain, numbness, a sense of pressure, stiffness, chills, flushing, spots, small discolorations, and color changes.

There are three phases in the historical development of the concept of points. In the earliest phase people would utilize any body location which was painful or uncomfortable. Because there were no specific locations for the points, they had no names.

In the second phase, after a long period of practice and experience, certain points became identified with specific diseases. The ability of distinct points to affect and be affected by local or distant pain and disease, was perceived as predictable. As the correlation between point and disease became established, names were assigned to these points. For example "wind pond" (Gall Bladder 20) was named because this is the site where flu or cold producing factors (wind) lodge in the body. When you have symptoms this spot is sore.

In the final phase, many previously localized points, each with a singular function, became integrated in a larger system which related and grouped diverse points systematically according to similar functions. This integration is called the "Meridian or Channel System".

6. Blood

In addition to being a substance, Blood is regarded as a force, a level of activity in the body which is involved with the sensitivity of the sense organs, as well as a deep level of the body in the progression of febrile (heat) diseases. Blood is manufactured in the Middle Burner (zhong jiao), using the Qi derived from the air in the Lungs and food digested by the Spleen. The major function of Blood is to carry nourishment to all parts of the body. It is therefore closely related to Nourishing Qi.

7. Qi and Blood

A good example of interdependence and the Yin/Yang theory are Qi and Blood. Ancient texts relate, "Qi is the Commander of Blood, Blood is the Mother of Qi." This is understood because Blood depends on Qi for its formation from air and food, and for power to move through and remain in the channels. Blood is the "Mother of Qi" because the strength of the Qi depends on the nutrition and moisture carried in Blood. The two qualities complement each other.

Problems with Qi are usually two types — Deficient and Stagnant
    Deficient Qi: seen as general fatigue, depression, pale complexion, swollen tongue,

and empty or fine pulses.

Stagnant Qi: occurs when Qi does not flow smoothly through the meridians. This creates dull pain without specific location, bloated feeling in the chest or abdomen, and possibly coughing or vomiting.

Problems with Blood are seen in two major types — Deficient and Congealed

Deficient Blood comes from blood loss, malnutrition, deficient Spleen energy (because this organ makes and controls blood), and Congealed Blood. General symptoms include: dizziness, pale complexion, dry skin, loss of hair (hair being an extension of blood), pale lips and tongue, and a fine pulse.

Congealed Blood comes from two distinct injuries to the Body. The first is damage to the body which stops the circulation of Blood. The other is chronic Stagnant Qi, when blood is not being moved through the vessels smoothly enough, and congealing results. Symptoms include: fixed (usually stabbing) pain, dark spots on the side of the tongue, hard swellings, and a rough pulse.

8. Essence and Spirit (*Shen*)

Essence is the characteristic of the body which is the basis for all growth, development, and sexuality. It is demonstrated in our constitution and condition.

Spirit (Shen) is the force behind one's mental state and actions. Thought, Emotions, and Consciousness are manifestations of Spirit.

9. Fluids

Essential for life are body fluids. They include: sweat, urine, saliva, tears and the various secretions. Thin secretions moisten the muscles, skin, flesh, and the membranes of the sensory and excretory openings. Thick secretions moisten and nourish the inner organs and brain, and lubricate the movement of the bones and joints.

10. Organs

The Asian concept of Organs is energy-based and therefore different from our western structure-based concept. In traditional medicine Organs are always paired. The Chinese call the relationship of the meridians and paired organs **Zang-Fu**. The Organs are divided into two principle groups: Solid and Hallow. Each solid Organ (Zang) has a mate, a hollow organ (Fu). One being more active and considered the husband, while the other is usually somewhat less active or receiving and is considered the wife. For example the Liver (solid - makes bile) is paired with the Gall Bladder (hollow - stores bile).

Zang organs produce, transform, and store the vital essence—Qi (Ki in Japanese). Fu organs serve as a passageway to receive, digest, and transport the nutrient essence within the body and to excrete the waste residue. The solid organ is more active and therefore considered more important to survival. It is also for this reason that much more is written about the functions of the solid organs.

ZANG (Solid)	**FU** (Hollow)
Heart (HT)	Small Intestine (SI)
Spleen (SP)	Stomach (ST)
Lung (LU)	Large Intestine (LI)
Kidney (KD)	Bladder (BL)
Liver (LV)	Gall Bladder (GB)
Heart Governor (HG) [Pericardium]	Triple Heater (TH) [Sanjiao]

Each organ has an area that is affected when disease is present.
- Lung and Heart show changes on the forearms
- Liver in the arm pits
- Spleen on the inside of the thighs
- Kidney at the back of the knees

Source of Blood

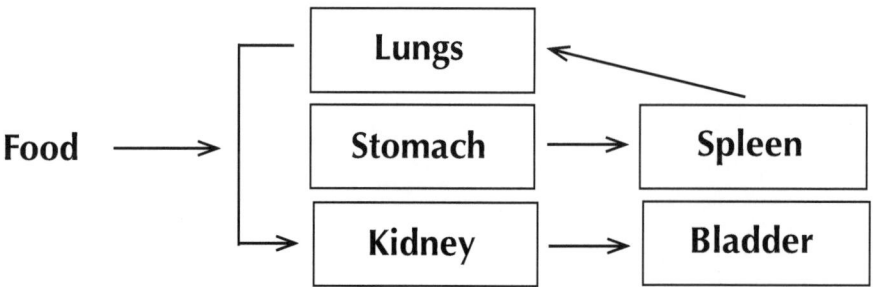

In addition to the material factors related to blood, we want to consider the energetic quality that blood has. In the ancient teachings there has been a strong connection between blood, body fluids, and energy. They are the essential substance within the human body. The body's energy is a reflection of the combined functions of the internal organs. This energy must be nourished by blood. The moisture of the internal organs is supplied by the body fluids. And the normal structure and function of the organs rely on energy. The production and distribution of energy depend on the normal physiological activities of the internal organs. These circular relationships of requirement and supply reflects the spiral nature of nature.

Blood originates through the transformation of food in the Stomach and Spleen area where it is received and digested. The essence that is extracted is transported up to the Heart and Lung areas. By the action of the Heart energy and the Lung energy it becomes blood. Food is the material foundation of blood. A secondary source of blood comes from the bone marrow, which is produced by the Kidneys. The Kidneys are regard as very important as they influence the energy of the Stomach, Spleen, Lungs, and Heart. The Heart and Lungs are responsible for the distribution of blood. This is accomplished by breathing.

Sources of Energy (Qi)

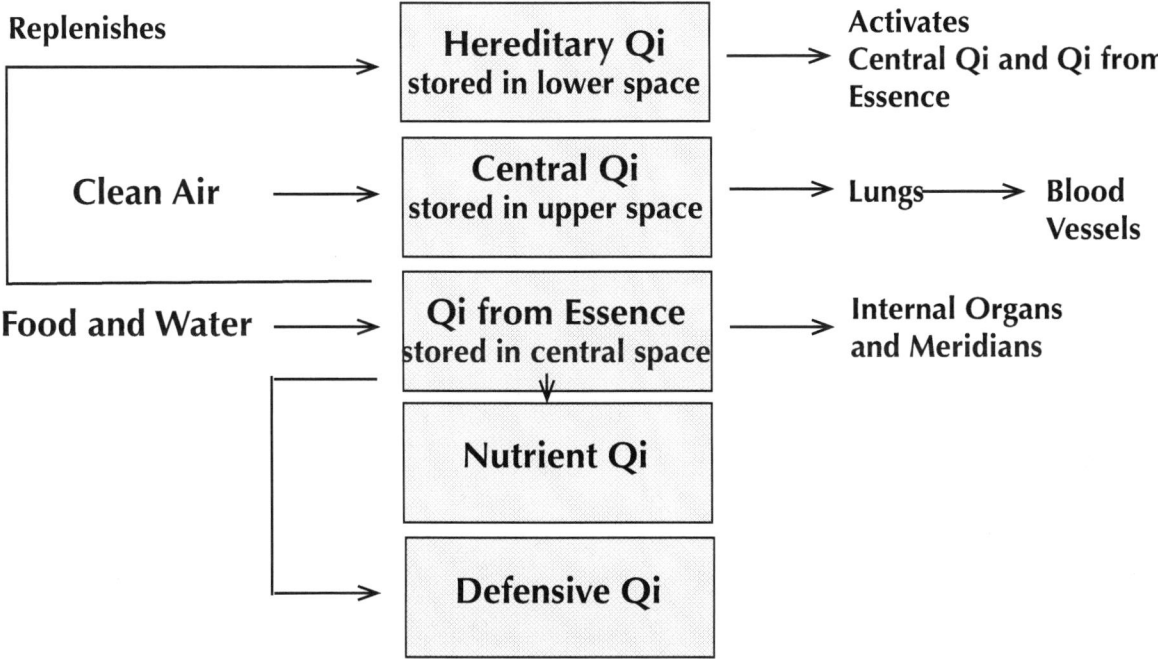

Hereditary Qi: primary Qi that is formed in the embryo. (*Yuan Qi*) After birth this hereditary Qi (non-renewable) continues to exist but it must be supplemented by Qi from breath and food. It is stored in the Kidneys.

Central Qi: produced by the combination of breathing "clean Qi" inhaled by the Lungs that is mixed with the Qi of food. Central Qi (*Zhong Qi*) is stored in the chest. It influences the blood vessels thereby promoting blood circulation.

Qi from the Essence of Food and Water: digested and absorbed by the Stomach and Spleen. This Qi is transported upward to the Lungs where it is mixed with oxygen (clean Qi) and becomes Central Qi. This Qi ensures normal life activities and provides the material source for these activities.

Nutrient Qi: supplies all internal organs with Qi to survive. Nutrient Qi (*Ying Qi*) also supplies the meridians with Qi. It produces blood and nourishes entire body.

Defensive Qi: this Qi (*Wei Qi*) flows outside the blood vessels, adjusts pores, and surface immune system. It protects and resists against disease.

Macrobiotic Shiatsu Workbook

Energy Flow Within the Body

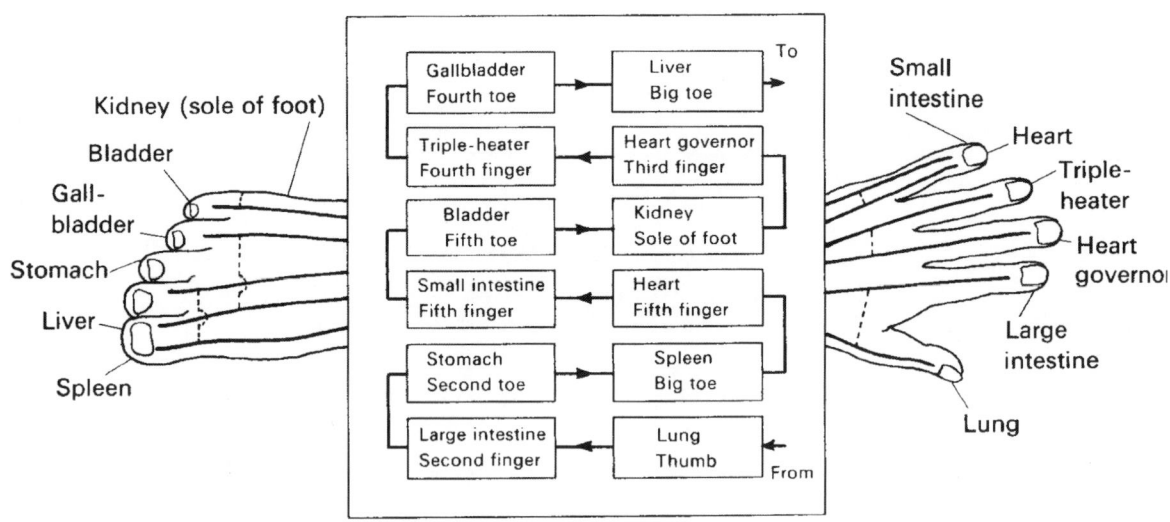

Spiral of Creation

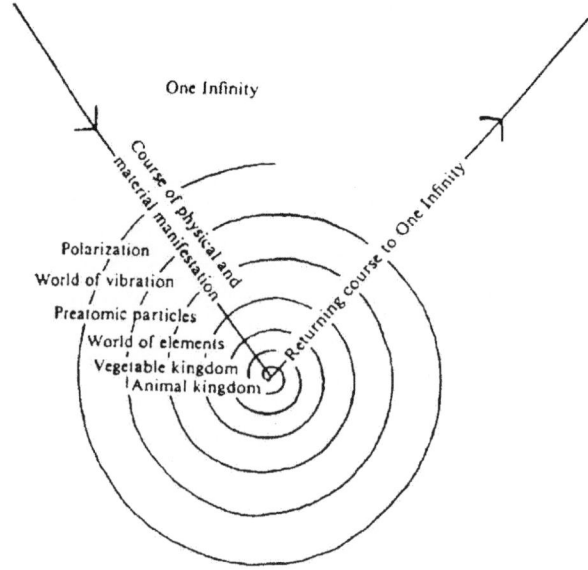

Face Diagnosis

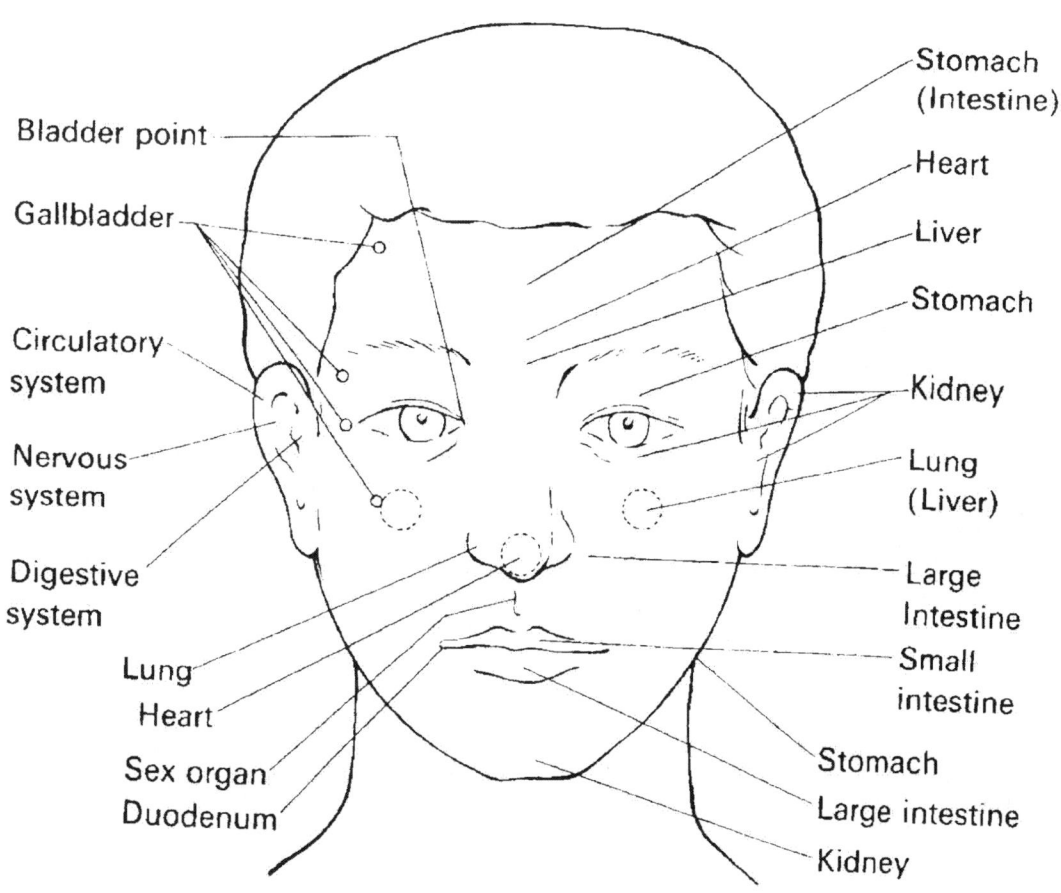

Macrobiotic Shiatsu Workbook

Internal Organs, Emotions & Facial Diagnosis

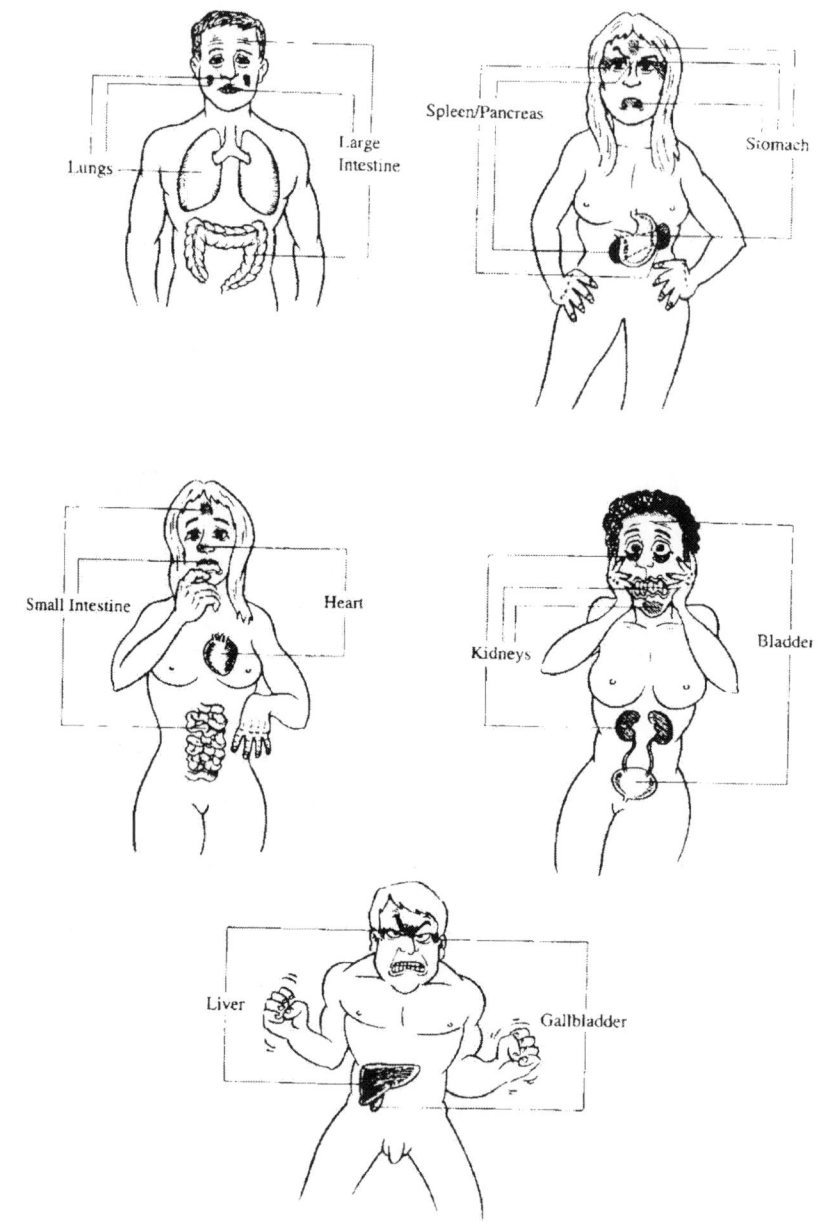

INTERNAL ORGAN	EMOTION -	EMOTION +
Lung / Large Intestine	Grief	Happiness/Security
Spleen / Stomach	Worry	Sympathy/Wisdom
Heart / Small Intestine	Excitability	Gentleness/Tranquility
Kidney / Bladder	Fear	Confidence/Courage
Liver / Gall Bladder	Anger	Patience/Endurance

Back & Front Points

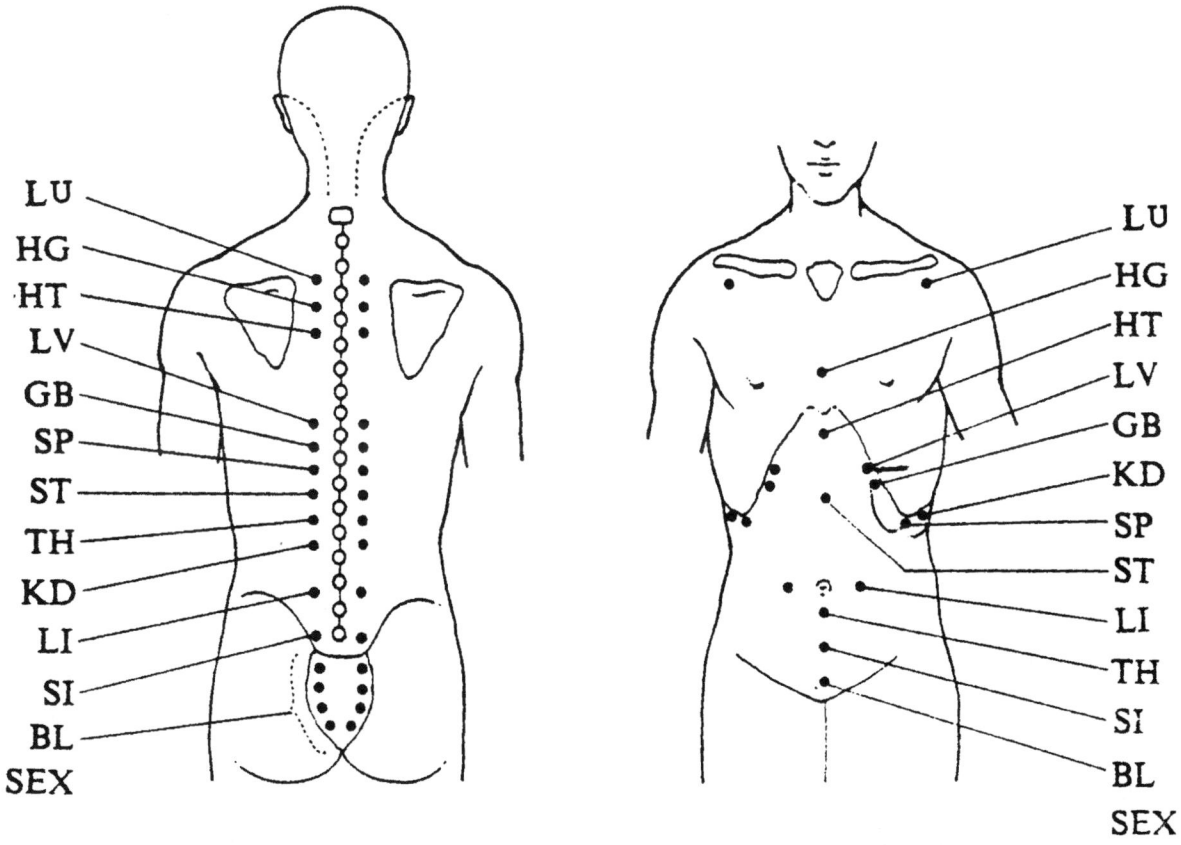

INTERNAL ORGANS	BACK POINTS	FRONT POINTS
Lung	BL 13 (Thoracic 3)	LU 1
Heart Governor	BL 14 (T_4)	CV 17
Heart	BL 15 (T_5)	CV 14
Liver	BL 18 (T_9)	LV 14
Gall Bladder	BL 19 (T_{10})	GB 24
Spleen	BL 20 (T_{11})	LV 13
Stomach	BL 21 (T_{12})	CV 12
Triple Heater (Sanjiao)	BL 22 (Lumbar 1)	CV 5
Kidney	BL 23 (L_2)	GB 25
Large Intestine	BL 25 (L_4)	ST 25
Small Intestine	BL 27 (Sacrum 1)	CV 4
Bladder	BL 28 (S_2)	CV 3

* Back Points are known as *Yu* points in Japanese and *Shu* points in Chinese.
Front Points are known as *Bo* points in Japanese and *Mu* points in Chinese.

Macrobiotic Shiatsu Workbook

Major Energy Centers — Chakras

Heaven's Force Enters Body from Crown

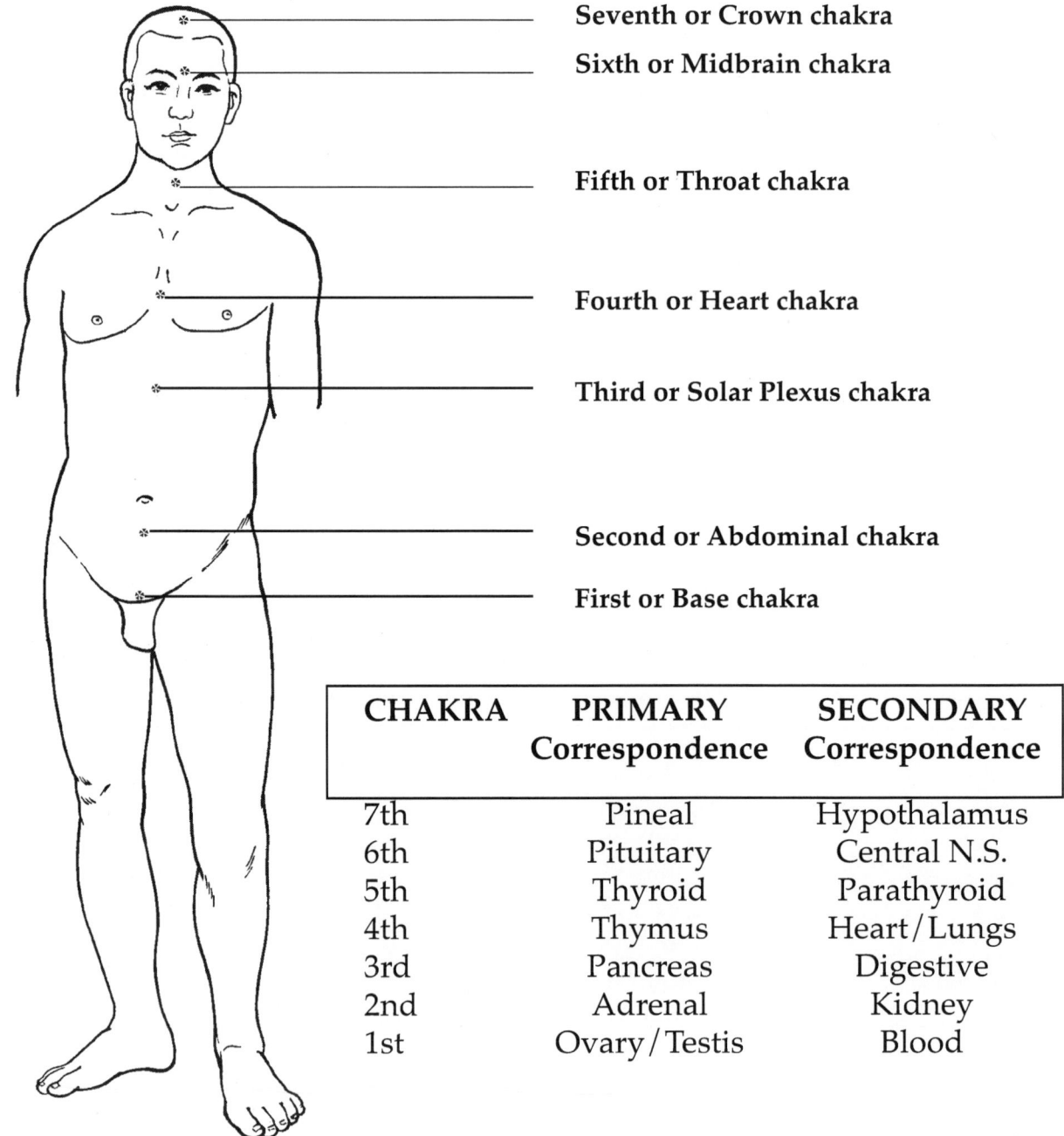

- Seventh or Crown chakra
- Sixth or Midbrain chakra
- Fifth or Throat chakra
- Fourth or Heart chakra
- Third or Solar Plexus chakra
- Second or Abdominal chakra
- First or Base chakra

CHAKRA	PRIMARY Correspondence	SECONDARY Correspondence
7th	Pineal	Hypothalamus
6th	Pituitary	Central N.S.
5th	Thyroid	Parathyroid
4th	Thymus	Heart/Lungs
3rd	Pancreas	Digestive
2nd	Adrenal	Kidney
1st	Ovary/Testis	Blood

Earth's Force Enters Body from Feet

Macrobiotic/Barefoot Shiatsu Techniques

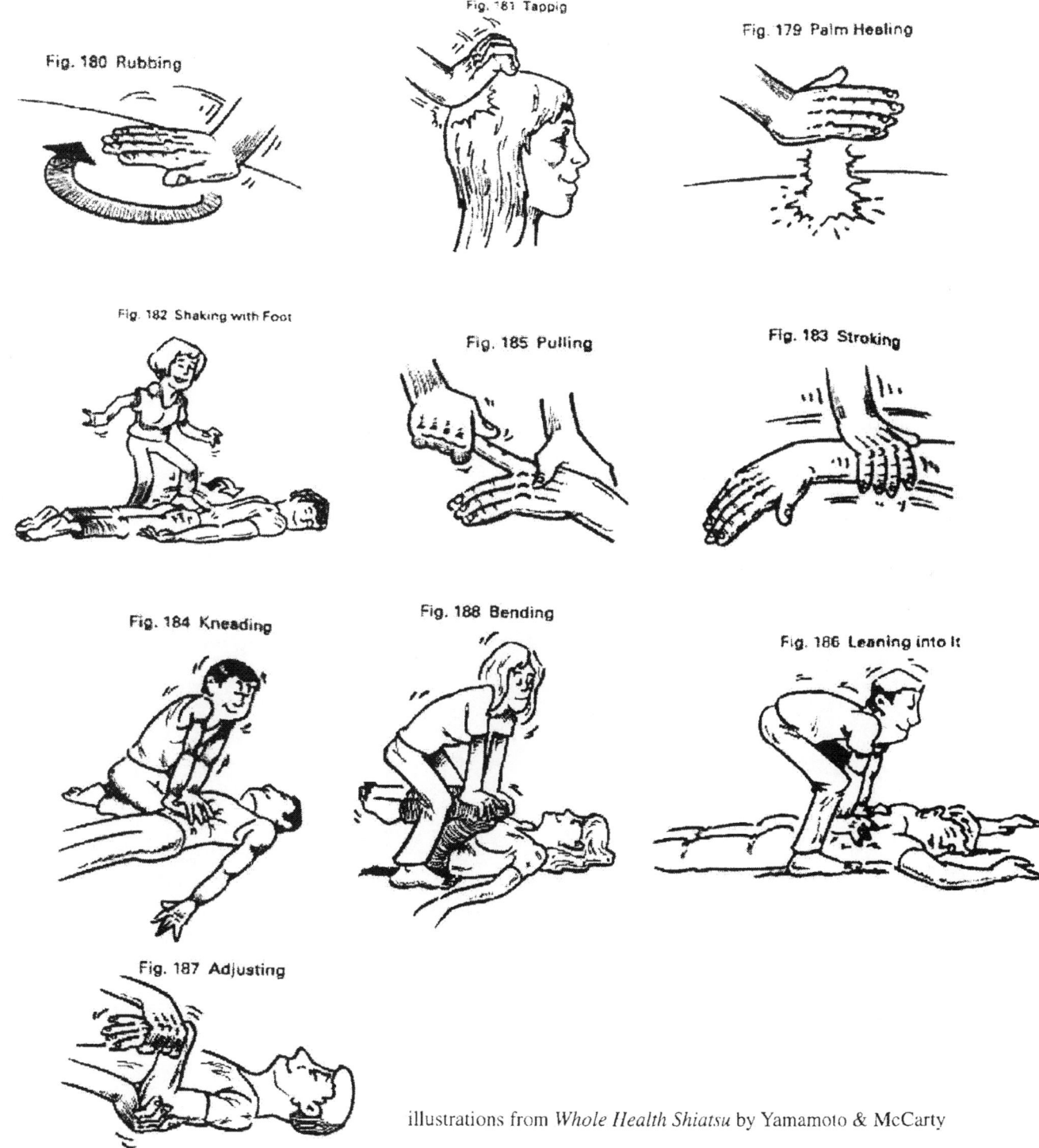

illustrations from *Whole Health Shiatsu* by Yamamoto & McCarty

Macrobiotic Shiatsu Workbook

Abdominal Organs

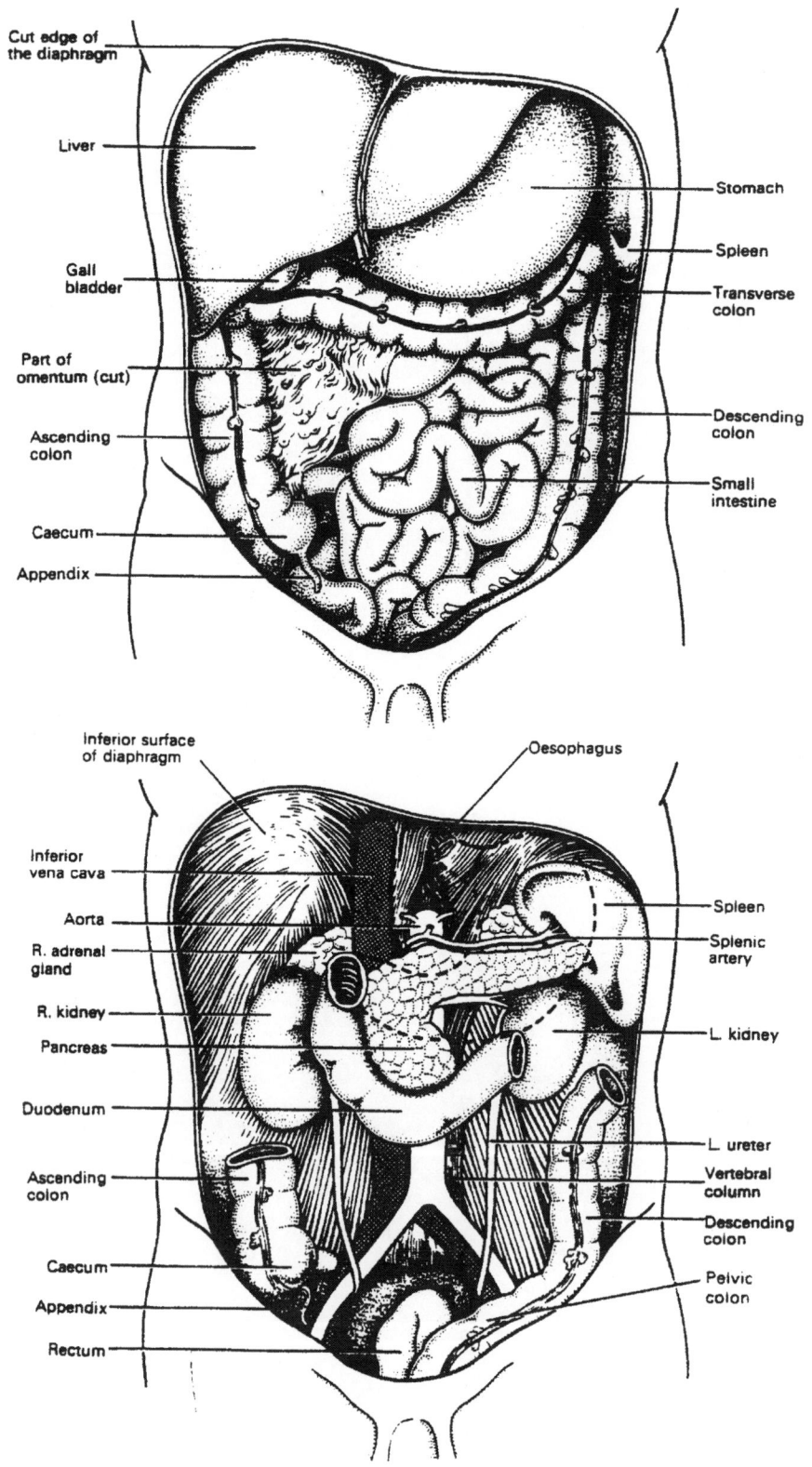

Macrobiotic Shiatsu Workbook

Macrobiotic Shiatsu Treatment

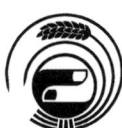

Barefoot/Macrobiotic Shiatsu takes between 45-60 minutes to complete a full session. The session is done with clothes on. Both practitioner and receiver should wear loose fitting cotton clothing. And throughout the treatment session both practitioner and receiver should coordinate the breath so both are breathing together. This strengthens the power of the session.

Basic Macrobiotic Shiatsu Steps

Receiver is seated on the floor or in a chair.

1. Loosen up shoulders.

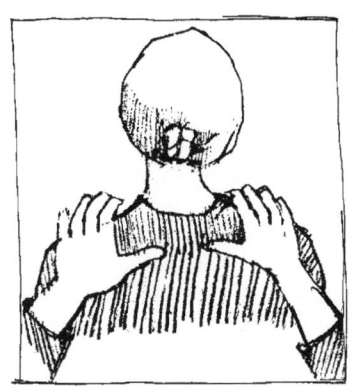

2. Pound across shoulders.

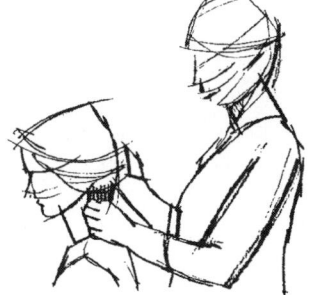

Receiver lies face down. Arms extended out at the sides, palms flat.

3. Foot on hip bone, roll the pelvis.

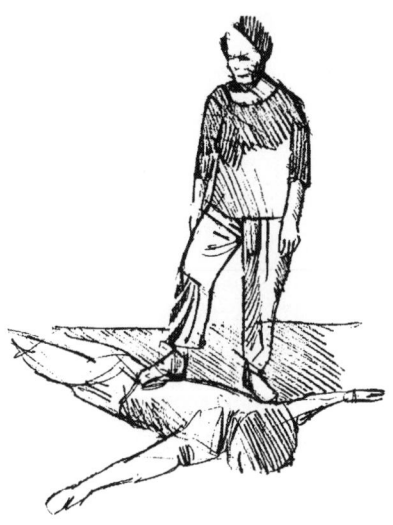

33

4. Walk on the feet. Sole to sole.

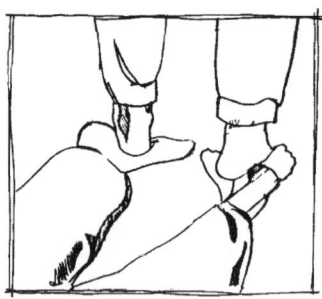

5. Foot presses the right buttock.

6. Foot presses the upper part of the right thigh.

Change sides and repeat. (numbers 5 & 6)

7. Stretch and rotate the arm.

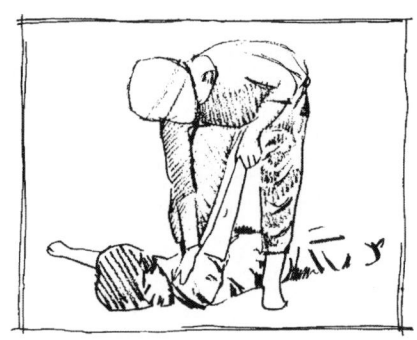

8. Arm up the back, press on the right shoulder blade toward the heart.

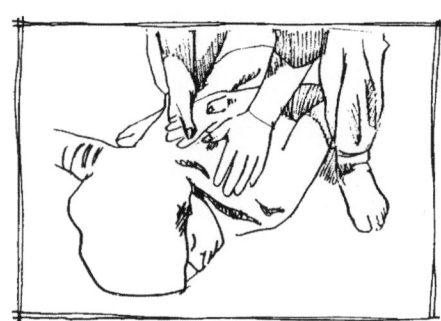

Change sides and repeat. (numbers 7 & 8)

Macrobiotic Shiatsu Workbook

9. Press down the back with palms flat.

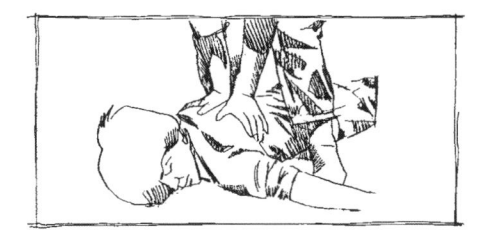

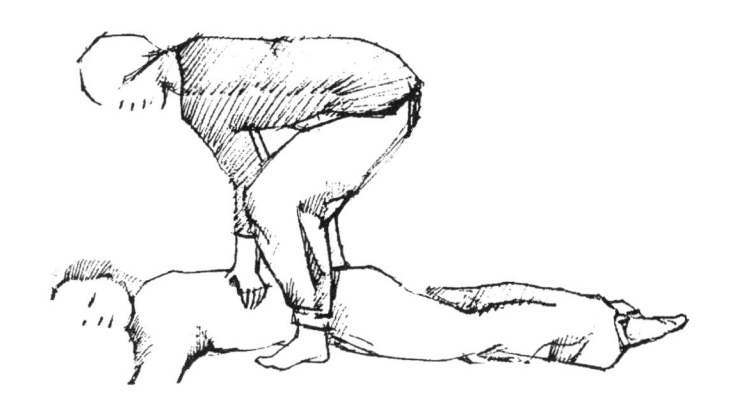

10. Press down the back with thumbs.

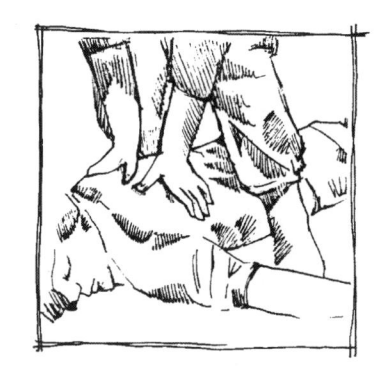

Move to the feet.

11. Press both feet down to the buttocks.

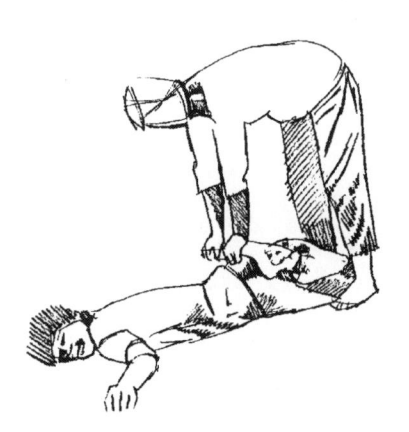

12. Cross legs and press toward the buttocks.

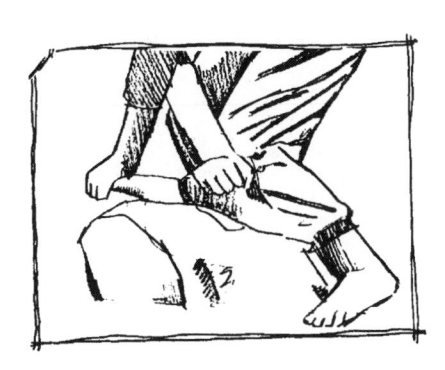

35

13. Pounding on the back with the fists and/or flat of the back of the hand.

14. Pick up one leg, walk to opposite side and stretch leg up while pressing on the back with your foot. Drop foot when finished. Repeat with other leg.

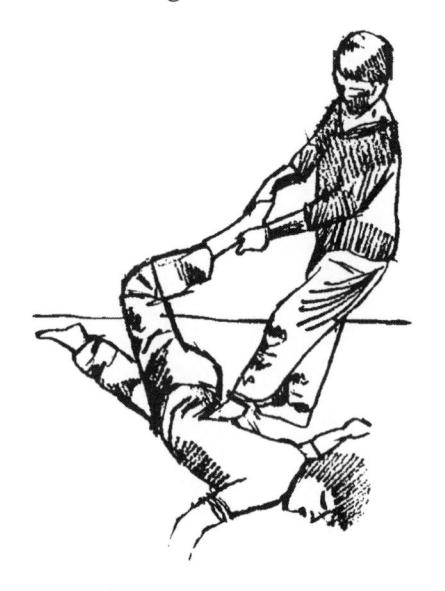

Receiver turns over.

15. Bring knees up together and bend toward chest on exhalation.

16. Rotate bent knees together in one direction then in the other direction.

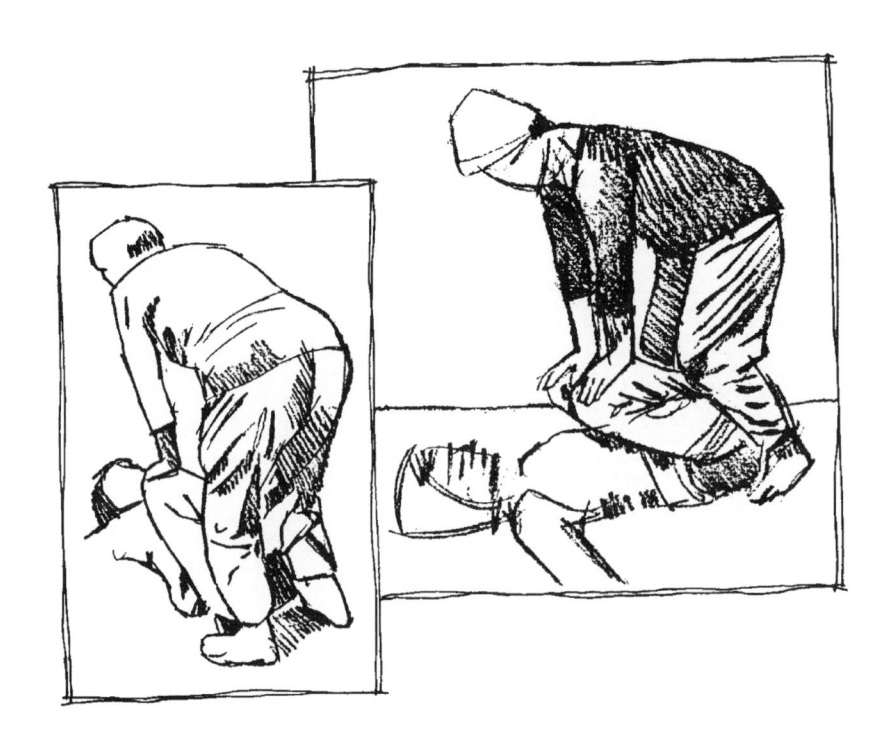

Giver moves to receiver's feet.

17. Pick up foot and brush toes with your hand, fingers pointing inward.

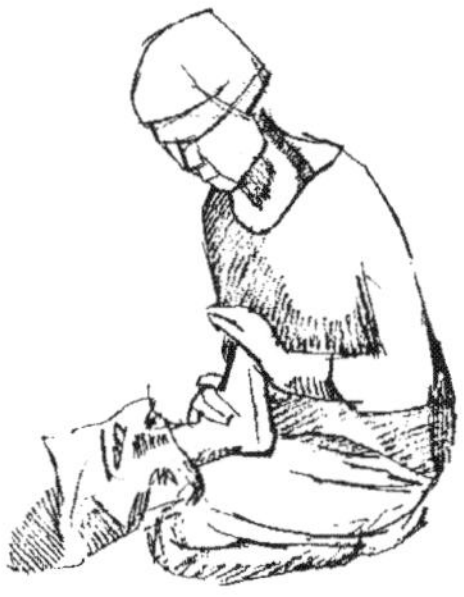

18. Press up outside of leg with thumb.

19. Press up inside of leg with thumb.

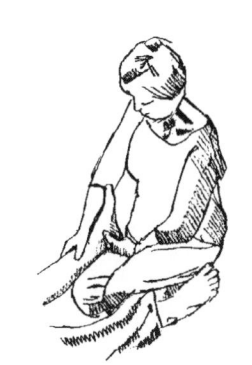

20. Manipulate each toe on the foot.

(Repeat on other leg. numbers 17-20)

Kneeling at receiver's side.

21. Both hands palms flat on lower abdomen, breathe together.

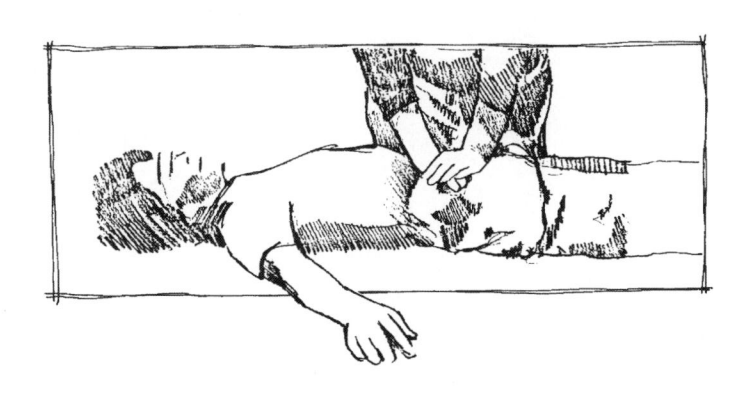

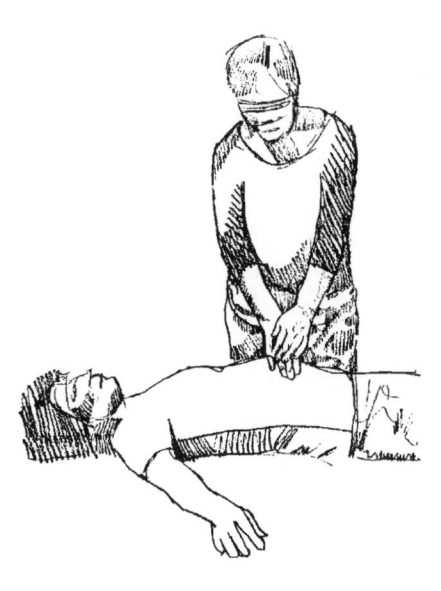

Giver moves to the hand.

22. Pick up hand, manipulate and adjust each finger.

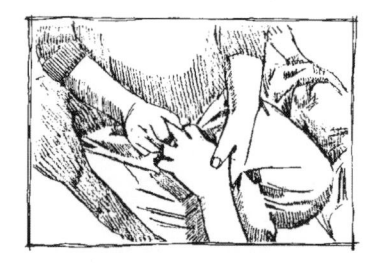

23. Place fingers between fingers and push back stretching fingers and wrist.

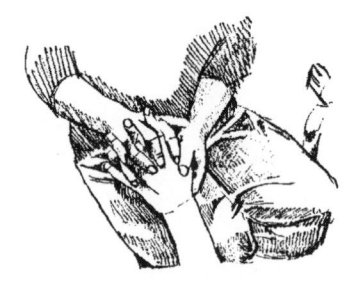

24. Press the center of the palm with thumb.

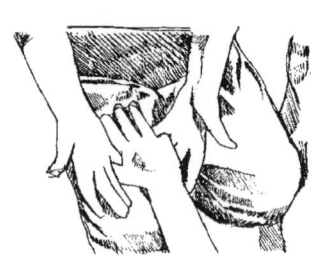

25. Press the upper arm with thumb.
26. Stretch arm outward and adjust the elbow.

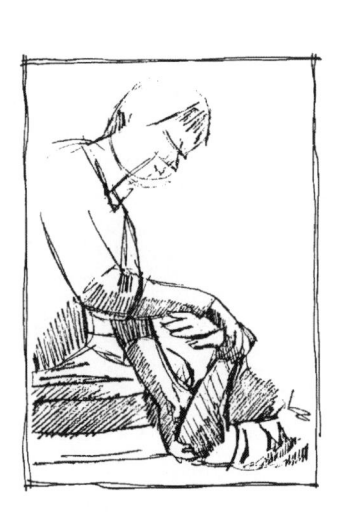

Move to opposite hand. (repeat numbers 22-26)

Move to head.

27. Pick up head and stretch the chin to the chest with exhalation.

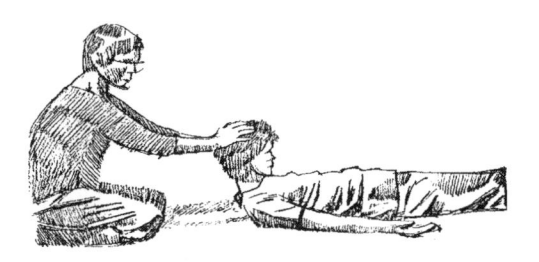

28. Hold neck on each side and pull toward yourself stretching.

29. Pick up head and rotate from side to side.

30. Press the center of head with thumbs together with vibration.

31. Press around the eyes, and on eye ball, cheeks, pull ears, base of throat, the sides of the chin.

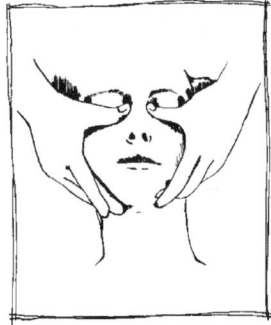

32. Pound the head with fist.

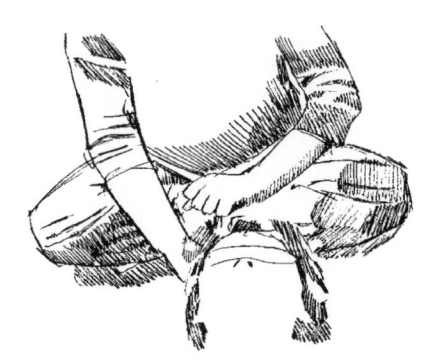

33. Hold head and breathe together several times.

END OF SESSION

Self-Shiatsu (Do-In)

Self-shiatsu is generally done in the morning. The primary purpose is to stimulate Qi throughout the body by directly activating the meridians. Treatment also breaks down any tension hardness and stagnation, while at the same time increasing circulation.

Take a comfortable sitting posture with spine straight and the shoulders relaxed. With the palms facing upward and resting on the lap, left hand on top of the right, close the eyes and meditate by simply releasing all thoughts. After several minutes in this quiet pose begin the Do-In routine.

General Order of Self-Shiatsu Treatment

1. With loose wrists and lightly closed palms, pound the top of the head in a counter-clockwise direction. Next, do the back and then the sides of the head.

2. Rub the ears vigorously, upward, outward, and downward.

3. Cup the right hand over the right ear and rhythmically tap the back of the hand with the left index and middle fingers. Repeat ten times.

4. Rub the face briskly, starting with the cheeks, then the forehead and finally the nose.

5. Massage the gums, top and bottom, with the tips of the fingers.

6. With the pads of the index and middle fingers resting lightly on the closed eyelids, softly press the eyes and release. Repeat ten times.

7. With the hands cupped over the eyes, look upward as far as possible, and then downward. Repeat ten times.

8. With the hands in the same position, look as far left as possible, and then as far right.

Repeat this sequence ten times. Then revolve the eyes in a clockwise circle and then a counterclockwise circle. Repeat ten times in each direction.

9. Gently rotate the neck in a clockwise and then a counterclockwise circle, three times each direction. Next, lightly pound the sides and back of the neck with the heel of the palm.

10. Pound the left shoulder with the right hand about ten times, then reverse shoulders.

11. With the hands and fingers, squeeze down along the arms, from the shoulders to the wrist. Start on the outside of the arm, then do the inside.

12. Press the back of the hand on a line from the wrist to the tip of each finger. Rotate each finger in both directions. Then massage the palm of the hand with lines from the wrist to the fingertips. Press the center of each palm with the thumb.

13. Lightly pound down along the chest, front and side, then down along the abdomen, front and side.

14. Bend forward and lightly pound the kidney region, then down the lower back. Stand and repeat on the buttocks.

15. Pound down the legs to the knees, front, inside, outside, and back. Then with the heel of the palm, rub from the knee to the ankle, front, back, and sides.

16. Rotate each ankle several times in both directions. Then press down over the top of the foot, on a line from the ankle to the tip of each toe. Rotate each toe in both directions.

17. Massage the bottom of the feet with the thumbs.

18. Stand and jump lightly about ten times. The shoulders and arms should hang loosely at the sides. Then repeat about ten times using only one foot and then the other.

END OF SESSION

Meridians

LUNG

In traditional Asian medicine, metal phase, the westerly direction, the season of autumn, the dry climatic condition, the color white, the emotions of sadness and worry, the pungent taste, and the sound of crying. It's opening is the nose, and it governs the skin.

The function of all organs in classical medicine is based on clinical observations of patients over hundreds of years and not necessarily the physical structure of the organ in western medicine. Most of the Lung functions have a common character: they are dispersing and descending in nature, that is they send energy away in different directions and especially downward. The Lung dislikes cold.

When a western anatomical description is explained the organ name is written with a lower case letter e.g. The liver filters the blood. When an Asian medical description is given the organ name is written with an upper case letter e.g. The Liver is responsible for an unrestricted flow of energy.

1. The Lung Governs Qi and Respiration.
The term "Ki" or "Qi" is often explained as vital energy. Although this term is not totally accurate, and there are different types of Qi, it is sufficient for this purpose. Governing Qi and respiration is the most important function of the Lung, because it extracts "clean Qi," energy from the air for the body, which combines with "food Qi," energy extracted from food by the digestive system. These two forms of Qi combine in the chest where they form Gathering Qi.

The Lung spreads this newly formed Qi all over the body to nourish the tissues and promote all physiological processes. This Qi also aids the Lung and Heart functions, as well as promoting good circulation to the limbs and controlling the strength of the voice. The strength, tone, and clarity of voice are all dependent on the Lung.

The Lungs are the most external of the Yang* organs, they are the connection between the body and the outside world. Therefore the Lungs are easily affected by exterior pathogenic (disease-causing) factors, and are vulnerable to invasion by climatic factors.

The Lung is classified as a Yang organ within Macrobiotic teaching (as well as Spleen, Kidney, Heart, and Liver). They are considered Yin organs by classical Asian Medicine. Both philosophies considered these organs to be solid.

2. The Lungs Control Pathways and Blood Vessels.

While the Heart controls the blood vessels in traditional Asian medicine, the Lungs play an important part in maintaining their health. The pathways refer to where energy flows in the meridians that help nourish the vessels along with the blood flowing with them. When the Lung Qi is strong, the circulation of Qi and Blood will be strong, so the limbs will be warm. While if it is weak, the limbs, especially the hands will be cold.

3. The Lungs Control Dispersing and Descending.

The Lungs have the function of dispersing Defensive Qi and body fluids all over the body to the space between skin and muscles. This ensures that ones resistance to external illness is equally distributed all over the body under the skin, performing its function of warming the skin and muscles and protecting the body from external pathogenic factors. A common cold usually manifests as an impairment of the Lung dispersing action. If this defensive energy is chronically weak there are exercises, foods and herbs that can build up the body's strength.

The Lungs have a descending function because the Lungs are the uppermost organ in the body. The Lung Qi descends to interact with the Kidney, while the Lungs direct fluids down to the Kidneys and the Bladder. If this function is impaired, cough, breathlessness, and stuffiness of the chest may result.

4. The Lungs Regulate Water Passages.

After receiving refined fluids from the digestive process, the Lungs spread them throughout the body in the area under the skin and controlling the bodies fluid loss through sweating. The Lungs also direct fluids down to the Kidneys and Bladder. An impaired Lung function could result in urinary retention.

5. The Lungs Control Skin and Hair.

The fluids that the Lungs receive from the digestive process and spread throughout the body under the skin gives the skin and hair nourishment. Thus if the Lung function is normal, the skin will have luster, the hair will be glossy, and the opening and closing of the pores and sweating will be normal. Also if this function of the Lung is impaired, besides affecting the quality of the skin and hair, the pores are often open with symptoms of spontaneous sweating. A person with these symptoms is often more vulnerable to attack from external disease causing factors, like catching a cold.

6. The Lungs Open Into the Nose.

It is said that the nose is the opening of the Lungs to the outside world. If the Lung Qi is weak, or if the Lungs are invaded by an external pathogenic factor, the nose will be blocked, and there may be loss of the sense of smell and sneezing.

Diet

Excessive consumption of cold and raw foods is said to affect the Spleen causing it to generate Phlegm that ends up being store in the Lungs. An excessive consumption of milk, cheese, butter, and other dairy products can have the same effect on the Lungs.

Emotions

The emotions that can effect the Lungs if they persist over a long period of time are sadness and worry. Prolong sadness disperses Qi, which results in a deficiency of Lung Qi. Prolonged worry causes stagnation of Qi in the chest that affects the Lungs.

Posture

Sitting for long periods of time over a desk to read or write can weaken Lung Qi, because the chest is impeded and proper breathing is impaired.

The Lung Meridian of the Hand (Yin Meridian)

There are 11 points on the Lung meridian. The Lung Meridian pertains to the Lung and communicates with the Large Intestine through the diaphragm. The meridian also associates itself with the Stomach and the Kidney.

Symptoms and Signs

External—Meridian: chills, fever, hidrosis or anhidrosis, nasal obstruction, headache, pain in the chest or of the shoulder and the back, decrease in temperature, and pain of the forearm and the hand.

Internal—Organ: cough, asthma, dyspnea (difficulty breathing), fullness of the chest, expectoration, dryness of the throat, color changing of the urine, increase in temperature of the palm, distress or hemoptysis (vomiting blood), accompanying occasionally with fullness of the abdomen and mild diarrhea.

LUNG MERIDIAN

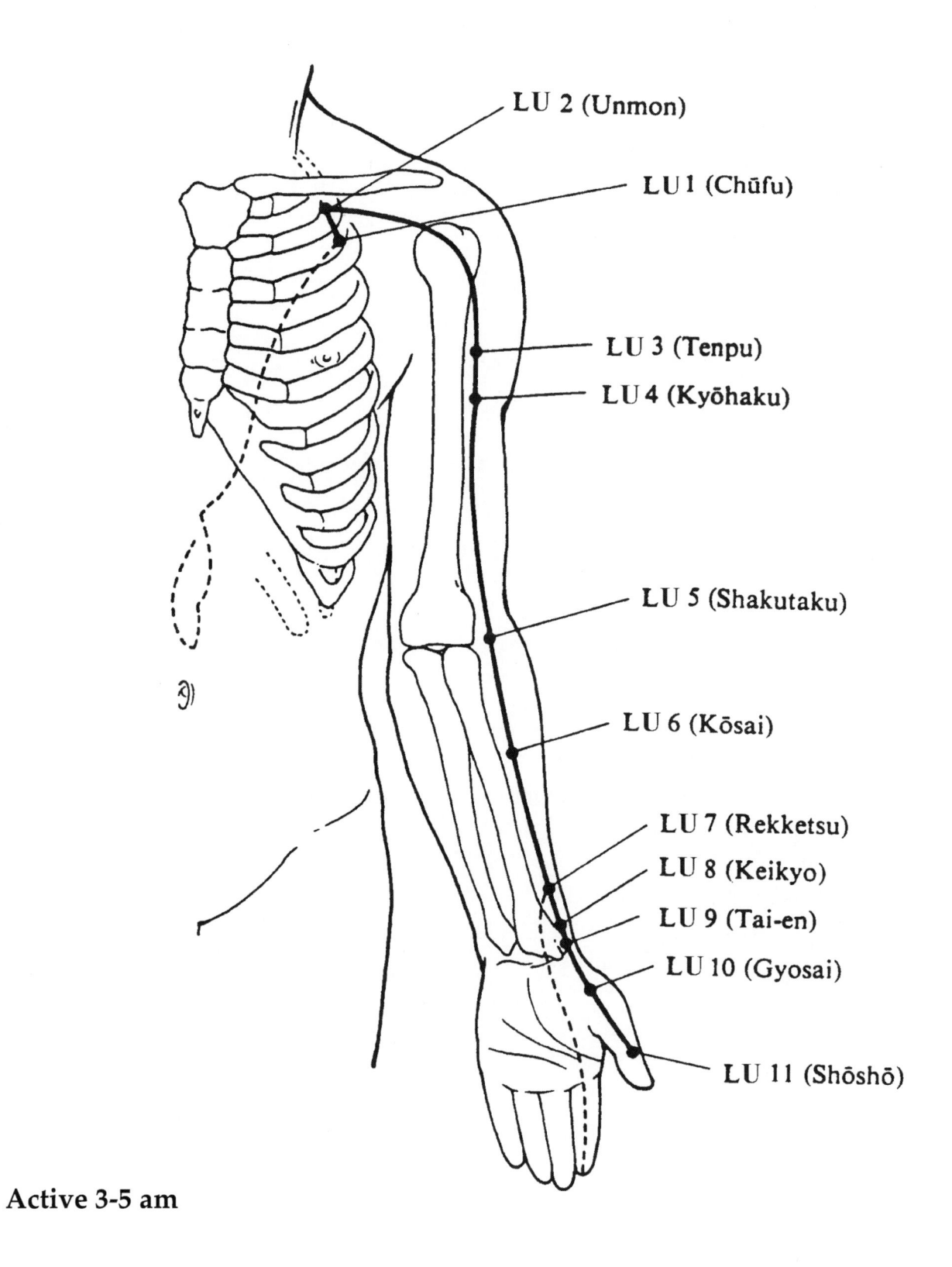

LU 2 (Unmon)
LU 1 (Chūfu)
LU 3 (Tenpu)
LU 4 (Kyōhaku)
LU 5 (Shakutaku)
LU 6 (Kōsai)
LU 7 (Rekketsu)
LU 8 (Keikyo)
LU 9 (Tai-en)
LU 10 (Gyosai)
LU 11 (Shōshō)

Active 3-5 am

LARGE INTESTINE

The large intestine is located in the abdomen. The upper end is connected with the small intestine by the ileocecum and the lower end empties into the outside of the body through the anus. The main function of the large intestine is to receive the waste material sent down from the small intestine and, in the process of transporting this waste to the anus, absorb any valuable part of its fluid content and then turn it into feces to be excreted by the body. The Large Intestine function can be summarized as that of transportation and transformation, typical of all Fu (hollow) organs.

The Large Intestine Meridian of the Hand (Yang Meridian)

There are 20 points on this meridian. This meridian pertains to the Large Intestine, communicating with the Lung and connects with the Stomach directly.

Symptoms and Signs

External—Meridian: fever, thirst, sore throat, epistaxis (nose bleed), toothache, redness and pain of the eye, swelling of the neck, pain of shoulder and the upper arm either redness and burning sensation or chills, finger trouble.

Internal—Organ: pain of the umbilicus region or abdominal wandering pain, borborygmus (growling stomach sounds), loose stools with yellowish mucus or complicated with dyspnea (difficulty breathing).

Large Intestine

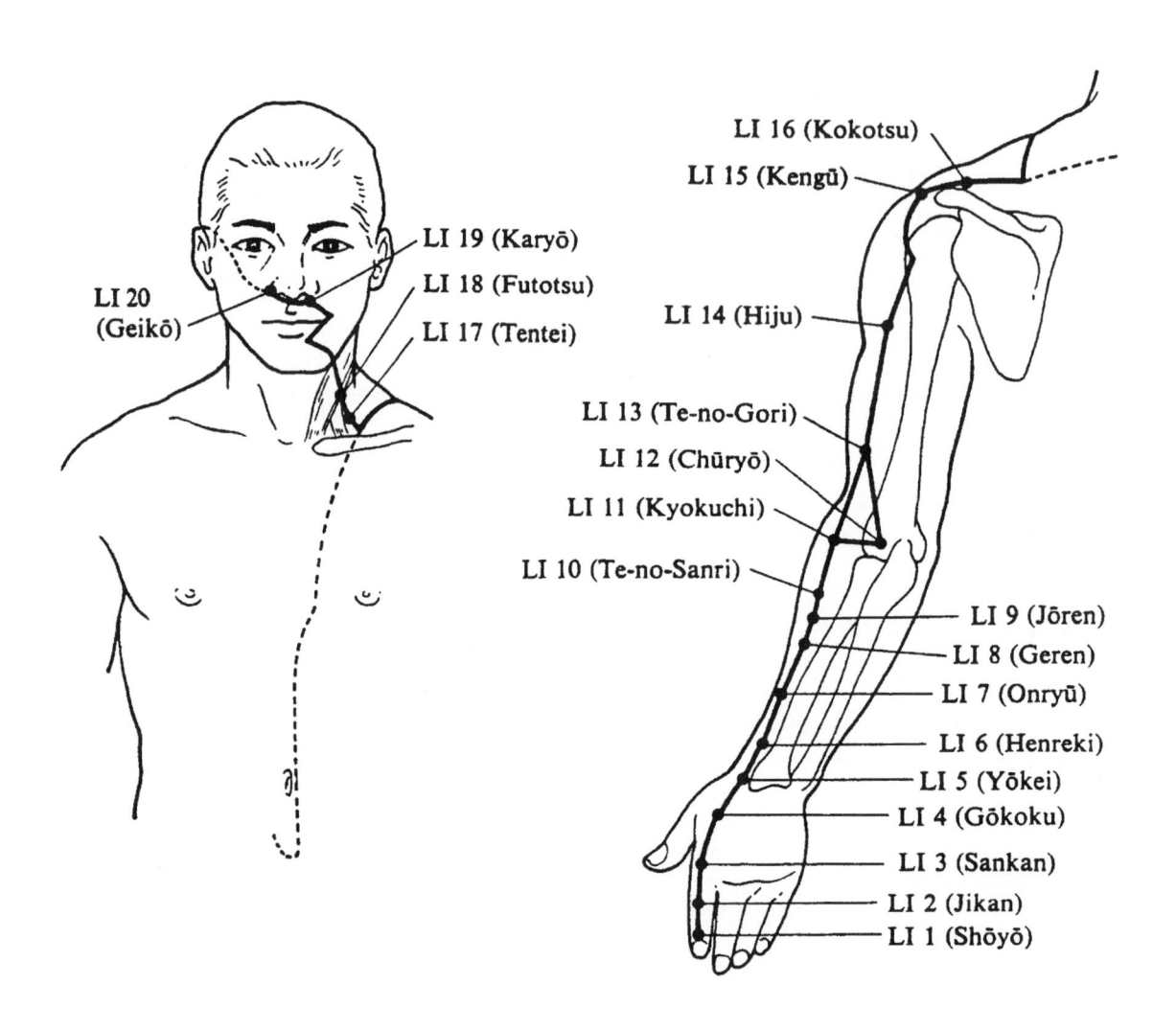

LI 20 (Geikō)
LI 19 (Karyō)
LI 18 (Futotsu)
LI 17 (Tentei)
LI 16 (Kokotsu)
LI 15 (Kengū)
LI 14 (Hiju)
LI 13 (Te-no-Gori)
LI 12 (Chūryō)
LI 11 (Kyokuchi)
LI 10 (Te-no-Sanri)
LI 9 (Jōren)
LI 8 (Geren)
LI 7 (Onryū)
LI 6 (Henreki)
LI 5 (Yōkei)
LI 4 (Gōkoku)
LI 3 (Sankan)
LI 2 (Jikan)
LI 1 (Shōyō)

Active 5-7 am

SPLEEN

The Spleen corresponds to the earth phase, the center direction, the season of late summer, the damp climatic condition, the color yellow, the emotions of anxiety and worry, the sweet taste, and the sound of singing. It's opening is the mouth, and it governs the flesh and muscles. The Spleen disperses energy upward and dislikes damp.

1. The Spleen Governs Transportation and Transformation.
The Spleen has the function of digesting food, absorbing its essential substances with a part of the fluid supplied, and transmitting them to the heart and the lung from where they are sent to nourish the whole body. Normal functioning of the Spleen is required for good appetite, normal digestion and absorption, good nourishment and normal transmission of fluid.

2. The Spleen Controls Blood.
The Spleen has the function of preventing blood from escaping the organs and vessels where it is supposed to be. It has failed in this job when excessive bleeding during menstruation takes place or nosebleed.

3. The Spleen Dominates the Muscles.
Strong muscles provide powerful movement and the four limbs will feel warm. The Spleen enables muscles to receive adequate nourishment from food essentials thereby maintaining muscle thickness and strength. Problems in this function result in weak muscles, cold limbs, fatigue, and atrophy.

4. The Spleen Keeps Organs in Place.
The Qi of the Spleen has the function of holding and keeping the internal organs in their

normal positions. When the stomach, bladder, or uterus drops the Spleen is failing in this job.

5. The Spleen Opens into the Mouth.

The Spleen function shows itself on the lips. The Spleen Qi passes through the mouth. This is how it influences the taste. The Spleen and mouth coordinate in receiving, transforming, and transporting food.

The Spleen Meridian of the Foot (Yin Meridian)

There are 21 points on the Spleen meridian. The Spleen Meridian pertains to the Spleen and communicates with the Stomach, then it connects directly with the Heart, the Lung and the Intestine.

Symptoms and Signs

External—Meridian: heaviness of the head and trunk, general fever, weakness of the extremities, pain of mandible and cheeks, tongue trouble, atrophy of muscles of extremities. Coldness on the medial aspect of the knee, and edema (swelling) of the leg and foot.

Internal—Organ: epigastric pain, diarrhea, indigestion, borborygmus (intestinal noises), vomiting, splenomegaly (spleen enlargement), loss of appetite, jaundice, abdominal distension, hard lumps in the abdomen, constipation, and dysuria (painful urination).

Spleen Meridian

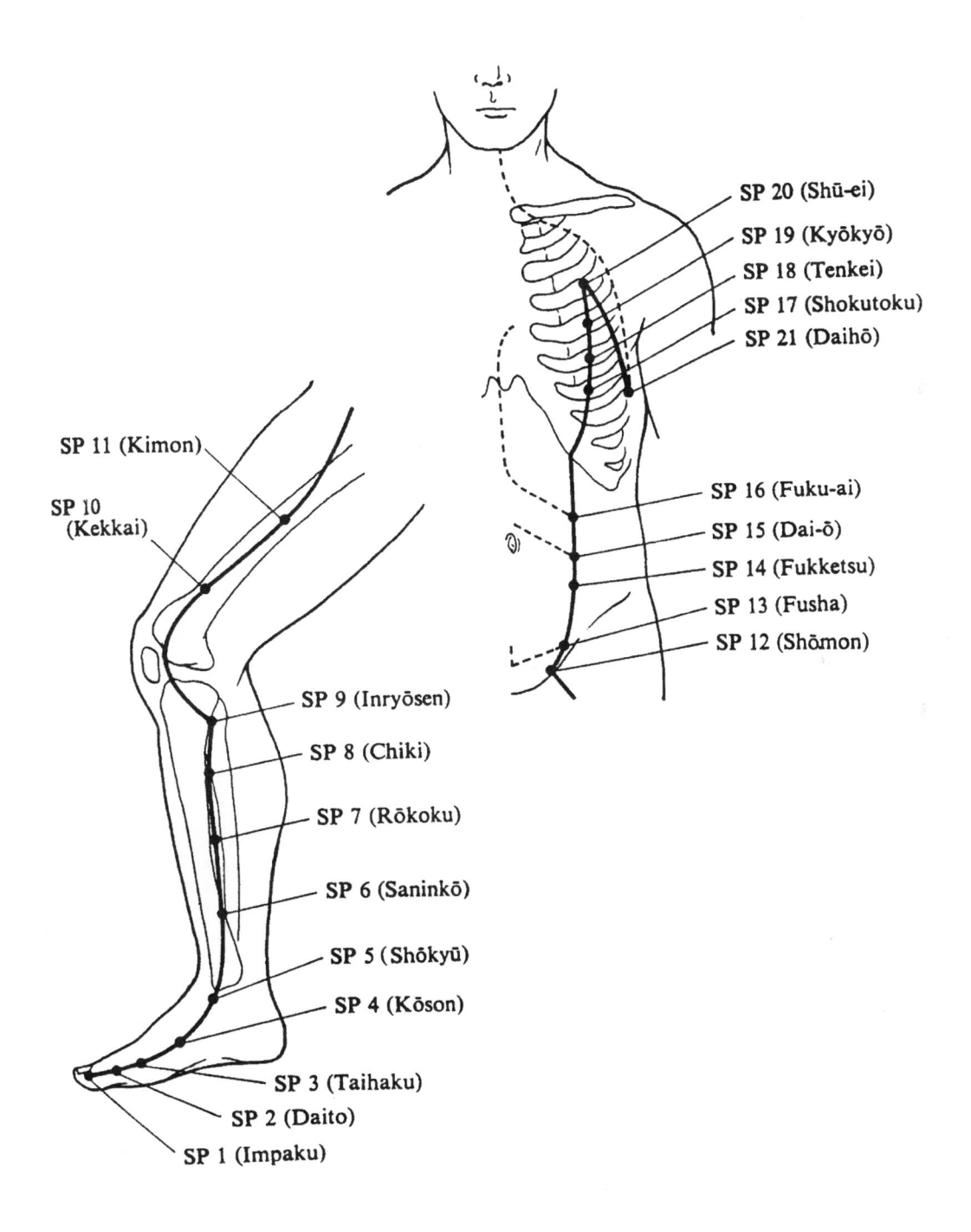

SP 20 (Shū-ei)
SP 19 (Kyōkyō)
SP 18 (Tenkei)
SP 17 (Shokutoku)
SP 21 (Daihō)

SP 11 (Kimon)
SP 10 (Kekkai)

SP 16 (Fuku-ai)
SP 15 (Dai-ō)
SP 14 (Fukketsu)
SP 13 (Fusha)
SP 12 (Shōmon)

SP 9 (Inryōsen)
SP 8 (Chiki)
SP 7 (Rōkoku)
SP 6 (Saninkō)
SP 5 (Shōkyū)
SP 4 (Kōson)
SP 3 (Taihaku)
SP 2 (Daito)
SP 1 (Impaku)

Active 9–11 am

STOMACH

The stomach is located close to the center of the body in the mid-truck region below the sternum (breast bone). The upper connection links with the esophagus and the lower outlet connects with the small intestine via the pylorus. Its main function is to receive and decompose food. The Stomach is called the "Sea of Food, Cereal and Water."

The stomach receives and temporarily stores the food mass coming from the mouth while partially digesting it and then sending it downward to the small intestine. The Spleen receives the nutrient essence from the Stomach and sends it to the Lungs. The normal function of the Stomach is to have a downward movement of energy. This force drives the changing food mass to leave the stomach and travel to the small intestine. When problems occur the Stomach Qi ascends rather than descends. This "adverse ascension of Stomach Qi" is seen as stagnation of food with its accompanying symptoms of abdominal fullness, distention, and loss of appetite. In severe cases there is vomiting, nausea, belching, and regurgitation of stomach acid.

Most of the stagnation disorders that occur in the Stomach can be attributed to excess. Overeating and the consumption of improper foods creates pain, burning sensations, irritation, bleeding, unusual hunger, halitosis and other troubles. Moderation and correct food choice remedies these situations. Because of the strong working connection between the Stomach and Spleen with reference to digestion and absorption, it is said that these organs are the source of health.

The Stomach Meridian of the Leg (Yang Meridian)

There are 45 points on this meridian. This meridian pertains to the Stomach, communicating with the Spleen and connects directly with the Heart, Small and Large Intestines

Symptoms and Signs

External—Meridian: fever, perspiration, red face, cloudy consciousness, delirium, eye pain, dry nose, epistaxis (nosebleed), fever blisters, sore throat, swelling of the neck, deviation of mouth, facial paralysis, chest pain, swelling of the leg, and coldness of the lower extremities.

Internal—Organ: abdominal distension, edema, disturbance of sleep, manic psychosis, discomfort when reclining, rapid digestion, excessive appetite, seizures, and yellow urine.

Stomach Meridian

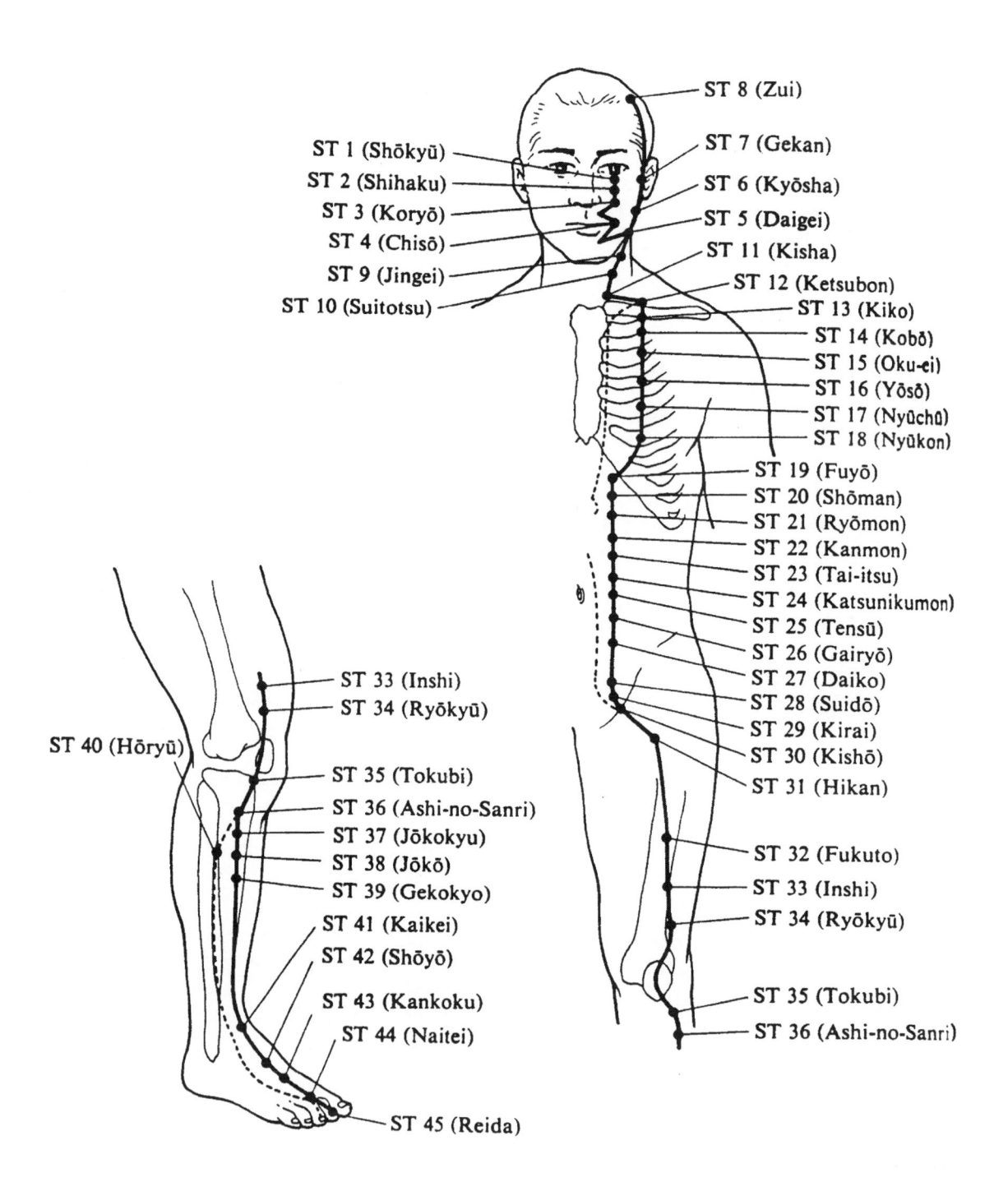

ST 1 (Shōkyū)
ST 2 (Shihaku)
ST 3 (Koryō)
ST 4 (Chisō)
ST 9 (Jingei)
ST 10 (Suitotsu)

ST 8 (Zui)
ST 7 (Gekan)
ST 6 (Kyōsha)
ST 5 (Daigei)
ST 11 (Kisha)
ST 12 (Ketsubon)
ST 13 (Kiko)
ST 14 (Kobō)
ST 15 (Oku-ei)
ST 16 (Yōsō)
ST 17 (Nyūchū)
ST 18 (Nyūkon)
ST 19 (Fuyō)
ST 20 (Shōman)
ST 21 (Ryōmon)
ST 22 (Kanmon)
ST 23 (Tai-itsu)
ST 24 (Katsunikumon)
ST 25 (Tensū)
ST 26 (Gairyō)
ST 27 (Daiko)
ST 28 (Suidō)
ST 29 (Kirai)
ST 30 (Kishō)
ST 31 (Hikan)

ST 32 (Fukuto)
ST 33 (Inshi)
ST 34 (Ryōkyū)

ST 35 (Tokubi)
ST 36 (Ashi-no-Sanri)

ST 40 (Hōryū)
ST 33 (Inshi)
ST 34 (Ryōkyū)
ST 35 (Tokubi)
ST 36 (Ashi-no-Sanri)
ST 37 (Jōkokyu)
ST 38 (Jōkō)
ST 39 (Gekokyo)
ST 41 (Kaikei)
ST 42 (Shōyō)
ST 43 (Kankoku)
ST 44 (Naitei)
ST 45 (Reida)

Active 7-9 am

HEART

The Heart corresponds to the fire phase, the southerly direction, the season of summer, the dry climatic condition, the color red, the emotions of excessive joy and excitability, the bitter taste, and the sound of talking. It's opening is the tongue, and it governs the blood vessels. The Heart disperses energy outward and dislikes heat. The Heart controls the blood vessels and is responsible for moving the Blood through them. It also stores the Spirit, and is therefore the Organ most frequently associated with mental processes.

1. The Heart Dominates the Blood and Vessels.

The Heart Qi has the function to prepare blood to circulate in the vessels. The vessels are the house for blood circulation. The Heart Qi must be sufficient or this will influence circulation. This can be seen on the complexion of the face. If the Heart energy functions well the person is full of vitality with normal pulse beats that are harmonious, powerful, and regular. If this energy is deficient then he tires easily. This function is viewed through the complexion and the pulse.

2. The Heart Houses the Mind.

Mental activity is involved with the Heart. "Spirit or *Shen*" is a general term of life activity of the body that can be seen by others. If there is abnormal Heart energy and deficient "spirit" then insomnia, lots of dreams, poor memory, restlessness, and mental disorders can be present.

3. The Heart Opens into the Tongue.

The tongue is the mirror of the Heart. Heart energy passes through the tongue and controls its color, form, motion, and taste sensation.

The Small Intestine separates the waste material from the nutritious elements in food.

The nutritious elements are distributed throughout the body, while the waste is sent on to the Large Intestine.

Almost all the disorders of the Heart are those of weakness.
Deficient Qi. General fatigue, panting and shallow breathing, and frequent sweating.
Deficient Yang. Swollen face, ashen gray or bluish-green, cold limbs.
Deficient Yin. Flushed feeling in the palms and face, low grade fever, & night sweating.
Deficient Blood. Restlessness, irritability, dizziness, absent mindedness, and insomnia.

The pattern Heart Excess arises from an excess of Heart Fire. This is marked by fever, sometimes accompanied by delirium, a racking pulse, intense restlessness, insomnia or frequent nightmares, a bright red face, a red or blistered and painful tongue, and often a burning sensation during urination. The later symptom is considered to be the result of Heat being transferred from the Heart to the Small Intestine, interfering with the Small Intestine's role in metabolism and the body's management of water.

The Heart Meridian of the Hand (Yin Meridian)

There are nine points on the Heart Meridian. The Heart Meridian pertains to the Heart connecting with the Small Intestine and has some connection with the Lungs and Kidneys.

Symptoms and Signs

External—Meridian: general feverishness, headache, pain in the eyes, pain along the back of the upper arm, dry throat, thirst, hot or painful palms, coldness in the palms and soles of the feet, and pain along the scapula.

Internal—Organ: pain or fullness in the chest and ribs, irritability, shortness of breath, discomfort when reclining, vertigo, and mental disorders.

HEART MERIDIAN

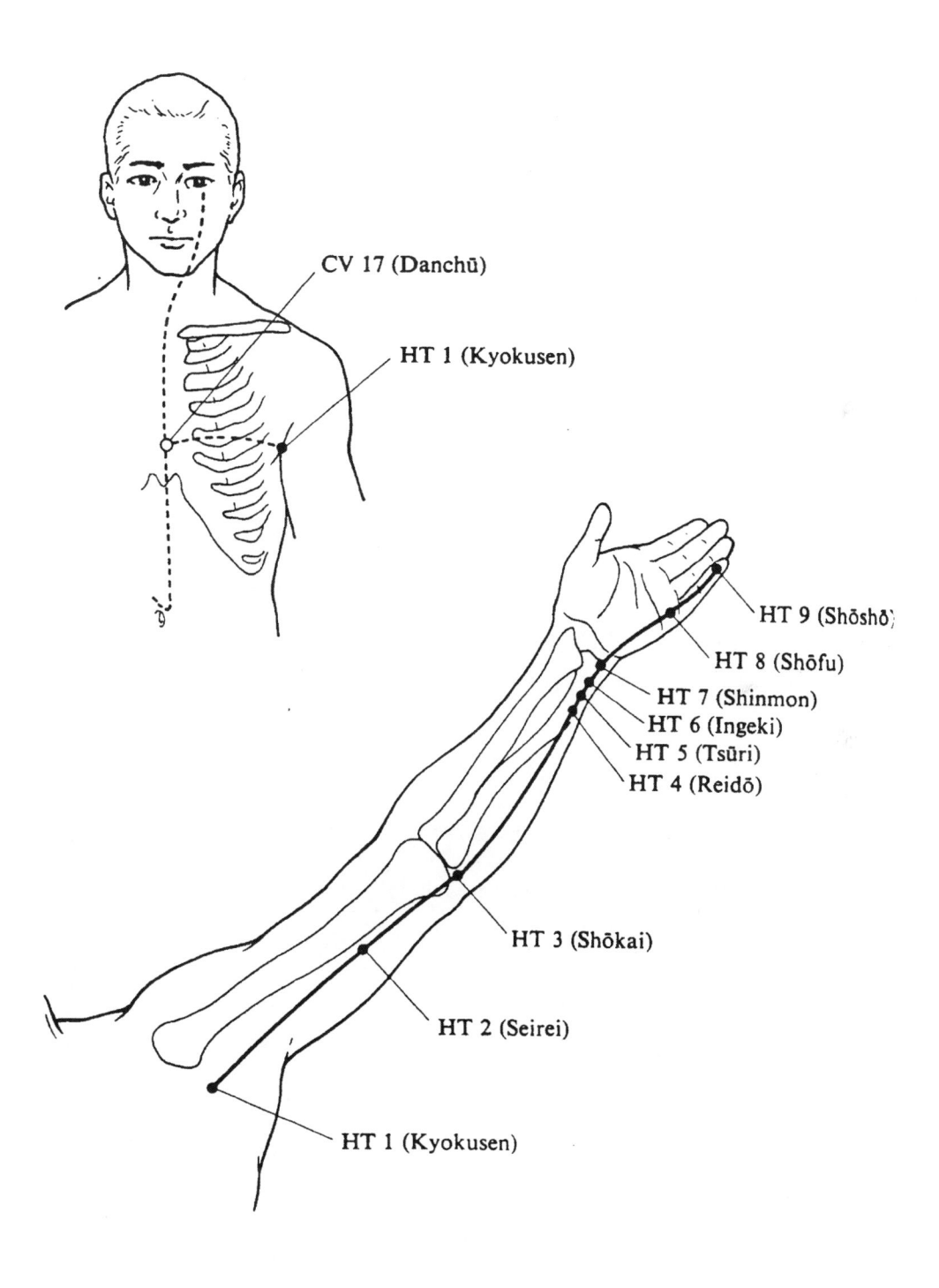

CV 17 (Danchū)

HT 1 (Kyokusen)

HT 9 (Shōshō)
HT 8 (Shōfu)
HT 7 (Shinmon)
HT 6 (Ingeki)
HT 5 (Tsūri)
HT 4 (Reidō)

HT 3 (Shōkai)

HT 2 (Seirei)

HT 1 (Kyokusen)

Active 11 am - 1 pm

SMALL INTESTINE

The small intestine is situated in the abdomen, its upper end connected by the pylorus with the stomach and its lower end connected with the large intestine through the ileocecum. The small intestine is an important site for absorption of nutrients that build blood. Its main function is to receive and temporarily store partially digested food from the stomach. It digests the food mass further and absorbs the essential substance and a portion of the water in food. The small intestine then transfers the residues with a considerable amount of fluid to the large intestine. In a similar way as the Kidney, the Small Intestine can separate essential from waste substance.

Problems in this function can be seen in the excretory processes especially in urination and feces production. Dysfunction stimulates urine to be plentiful while the stool may move excessively fast without time to have water soluble nutrients removed. This makes a soft or watery stool. The reverse can also occur and may create constipation. A hyperactive Small Intestine may be caused by Heart Fire that produces scanty red urine with a hot sensation during urination.

The Small Intestine Meridian of the Hand (Yang Meridian)

There are 19 points on this meridian. The Small Intestine meridian pertains to the Small Intestine connecting with the Heart and has some direct connections with the Stomach.

Symptoms and Signs

External—Meridian: numbness of the mouth and tongue, pain in the neck or cheek, sore throat, stiff neck, excessive watering of the eyes, and pain along the lateral aspect of the shoulder and upper arm.

Internal—Organ: pain and distension in the lower abdomen, possibly extending around the waist or to the genitals, diarrhea, abdominal pain with dry stool or constipation.

Small Intestine

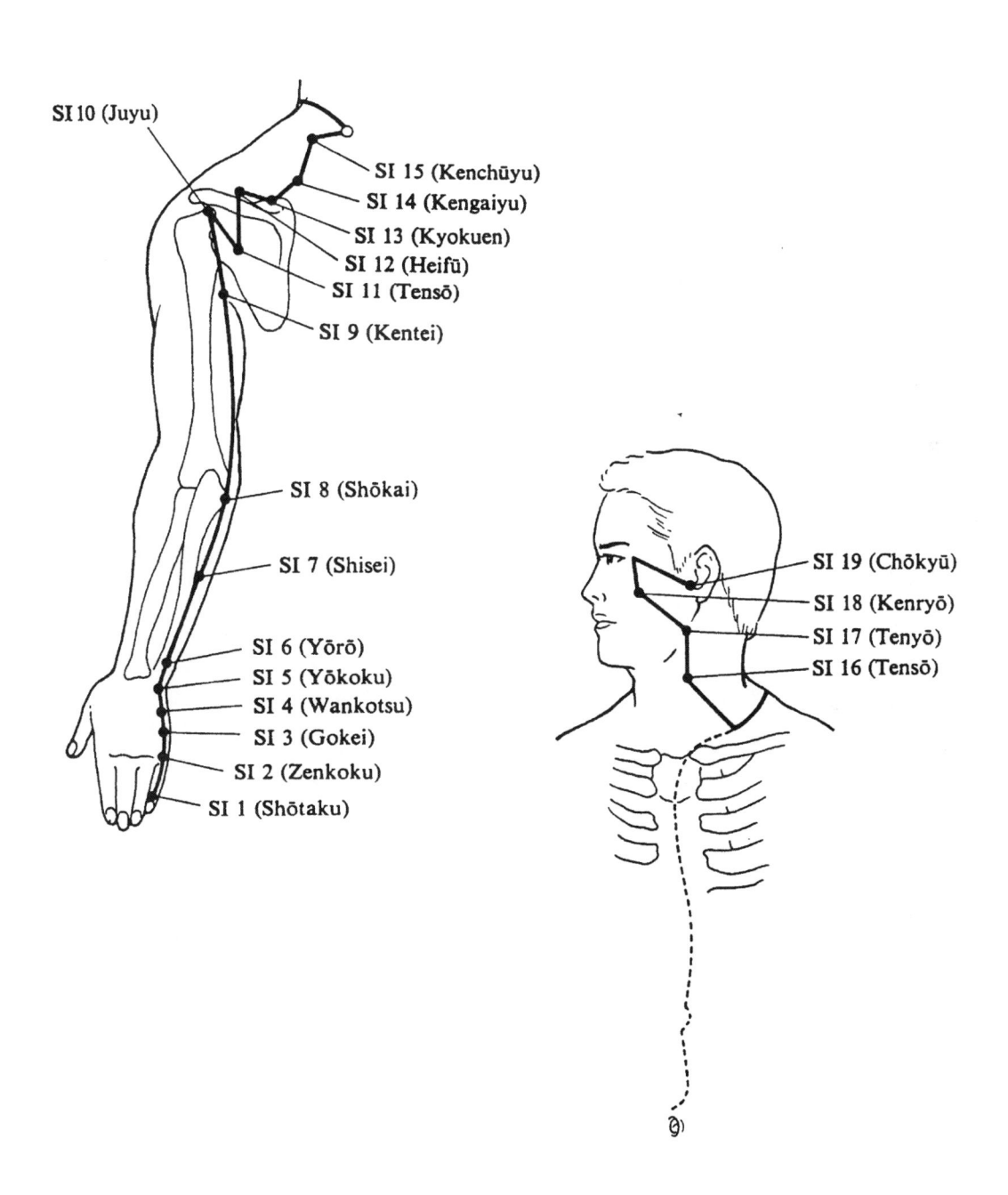

SI 10 (Juyu)
SI 15 (Kenchūyu)
SI 14 (Kengaiyu)
SI 13 (Kyokuen)
SI 12 (Heifū)
SI 11 (Tensō)
SI 9 (Kentei)
SI 8 (Shōkai)
SI 7 (Shisei)
SI 6 (Yōrō)
SI 5 (Yōkoku)
SI 4 (Wankotsu)
SI 3 (Gokei)
SI 2 (Zenkoku)
SI 1 (Shōtaku)

SI 19 (Chōkyū)
SI 18 (Kenryō)
SI 17 (Tenyō)
SI 16 (Tensō)

Active 1-3 pm

KIDNEY

The Kidney corresponds to the water phase, the northerly direction, the season of winter, the cold climatic condition, the color black, the emotion of fear, the salty taste, and the sound of groaning. The sensory organ is the ear. Their openings are the urethra and anus. They control the bones, marrow, and brain and their health is reflected in the hair of the head. The Kidney dislikes cold.

1. The Kidney Controls Growth.
The Kidney is the storage place for hereditary inheritance. The hereditary essence is the material foundation that allows the assimilation of acquired or replenished essence. Acquired essence is renewable and comes from food and drink. This energy must replenish the hereditary essence because only if acquired essence is present can development and growth take place. The Kidney also regulates growth of females at seven year intervals, while males are regulated at eight year intervals. Kidney energy exerts a strong influence at approximately fourteen years old with the beginning of the reproductive cycle and menstruation; at four times seven years, twenty-eight years of age, the physical prime of life is near a peak; and at age forty-nine, the cessation of menses and the child bearing years are over. For men, reproduction begins at approximately age sixteen; the prime of life occurs around age thirty-two (eight times four); decline begins at age fifty-six, and the ancients felt that by age sixty-four Qi declines to such a degree that the teeth and hair begin to fall out.

2. The Kidney Dominates Water Metabolism.
The three main organs involved in water balance are: Kidney-Lung-Spleen. The Kidney has the ability to separate the useful liquid from the waste and to send the useful up to the Lung (as moisture) and the waste to the Bladder (as urine). The Kidney first separates the clean from the turbid and then eliminates the waste.

3. The Kidney Dominates the Reception of Qi (Air).

The Kidney mainly receives Qi. It is also in charge of breathing. The distribution of the clean Qi inhaled by the Lung to the whole body depends not only on the descending function of the Lung but also on the Kidney's function of reception and control.

4. The Kidney Dominates the Bones.

Growth and development of bones comes from the Kidney essence. Kidney essence produces marrow. The upper part of the spinal cord connects with the brain, while the bone marrow nourishes the bones and manufactures blood. The supply to the brain, the solidity of the bone, and the adequacy of the blood are therefore all closely related to the condition of the essence of the Kidney.

The Kidneys are the storage place of basal Yin and Yang of the body. Therefore, any disorder, if sufficiently chronic, will involve the Kidneys. Diseased Kidneys will affect other organs.

Symptoms of Deficient Kidney Yin

The lower back is weak and sore, there is ringing in the ears and loss of hearing acuity, the face is ashen or dark, especially under the eyes. Dizziness, thirst, night sweats, and low grade fevers are common. Men have little semen and tend toward premature ejaculation, while women have little or no menstruation.
This deficiency produces similar disorders in the Heart and Liver.

Symptoms of Deficient Kidney Yang

This pattern is generally seen as loss of warmth along with the previously mentioned symptoms. There is a feeling of fatigue and coldness. There is a notable weakness of the legs. Excessive urination is also present. And sometimes faint voice, coughing, puffiness in the face, and spontaneous sweating.

This deficiency produces similar disorders in the Spleen and Lungs.

The Kidney Meridian of the Leg (Yin Meridian)

There are 27 points on the Kidney meridian. This meridian pertains to the Kidney to communicate with the Kidney and connects directly with the Liver, Lung, Heart, and other organs.

Symptoms and Signs

External—Meridian: back pain, lumbago, cold feeling in the feet, weakness of the feet, thirst, sore throat, pain in the back of the leg and thigh.

Internal—Organ: dizziness, facial edema, ashen complexion, blurred vision, shortness of breath, drowsiness, irritability, loose stool, chronic diarrhea or constipation, abdominal distension, vomiting, and impotence.

KIDNEY MERIDIAN

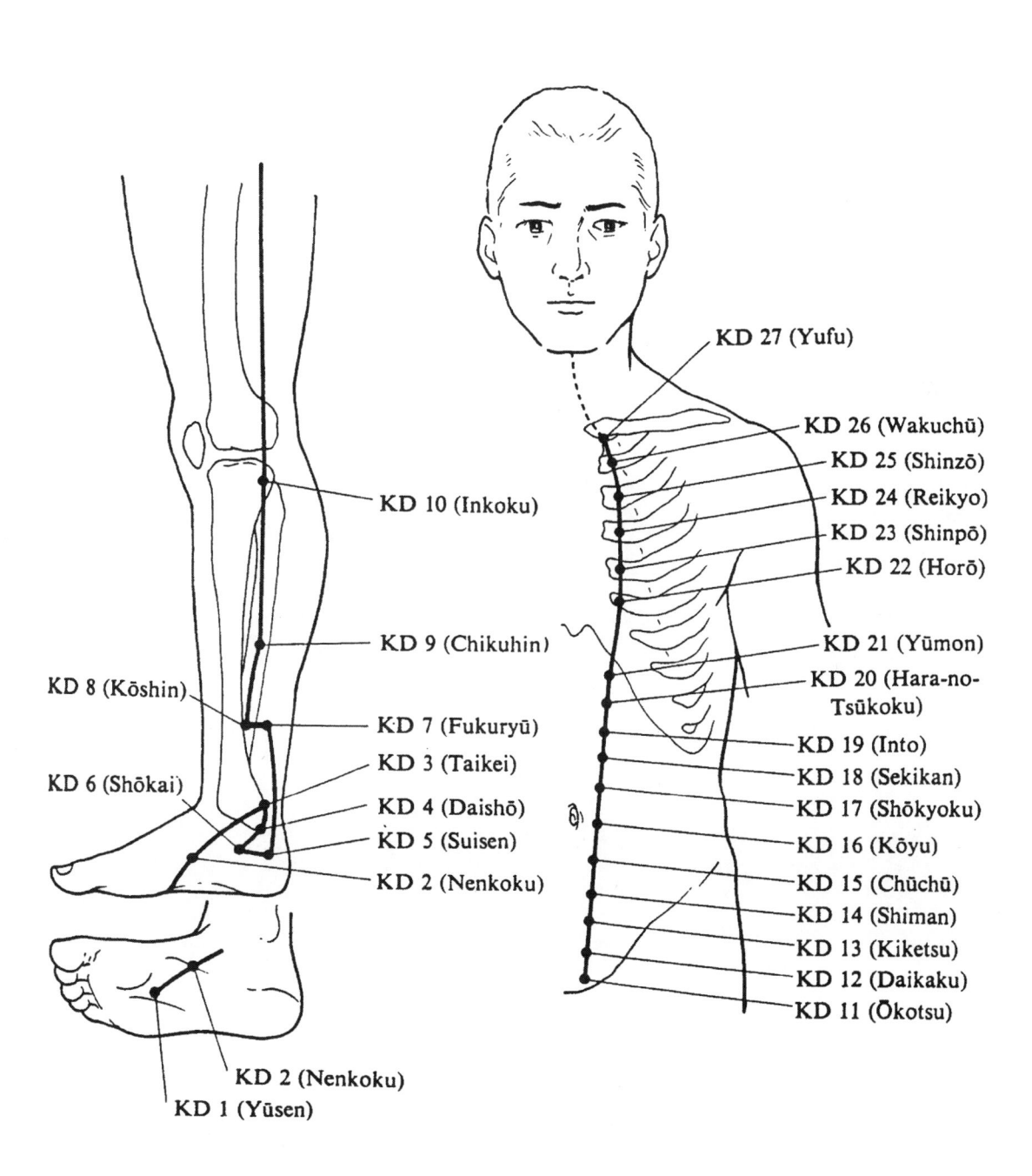

- KD 27 (Yufu)
- KD 26 (Wakuchū)
- KD 25 (Shinzō)
- KD 24 (Reikyo)
- KD 23 (Shinpō)
- KD 22 (Horō)
- KD 21 (Yūmon)
- KD 20 (Hara-no-Tsūkoku)
- KD 19 (Intō)
- KD 18 (Sekikan)
- KD 17 (Shōkyoku)
- KD 16 (Kōyu)
- KD 15 (Chūchū)
- KD 14 (Shiman)
- KD 13 (Kiketsu)
- KD 12 (Daikaku)
- KD 11 (Ōkotsu)

- KD 10 (Inkoku)
- KD 9 (Chikuhin)
- KD 8 (Kōshin)
- KD 7 (Fukuryū)
- KD 3 (Taikei)
- KD 6 (Shōkai)
- KD 4 (Daishō)
- KD 5 (Suisen)
- KD 2 (Nenkoku)
- KD 2 (Nenkoku)
- KD 1 (Yūsen)

Active 5-7 pm

BLADDER

The bladder is located in the lower abdomen behind and below the pubic bone. The main functions of the bladder are to receive, temporarily store, and excrete urine from the body. Urine is made by the filtering action of the kidneys. The Bladder function is accomplished with the help of Kidney Qi. All urinary problems are caused by dysfunction of the Kidney and Bladder.

The Bladder Meridian of the Foot (Yang Meridian)

There are 67 points on this meridian. The Bladder Meridian pertains to the Bladder connecting with the Kidney and has some direct connections with the Brain and Heart.

Symptoms and Signs

External—Meridian: alternating chills and fever, headache, stiff neck, lumbago, sinus trouble, frequent tearing, pain of the eye, thigh, back of the knees, leg, and feet.

Internal—Organ: lower abdominal pain, dysuria (painful urination), retention of urine, enuresis (bed-wetting), and mental disorders.

BLADDER MERIDIAN

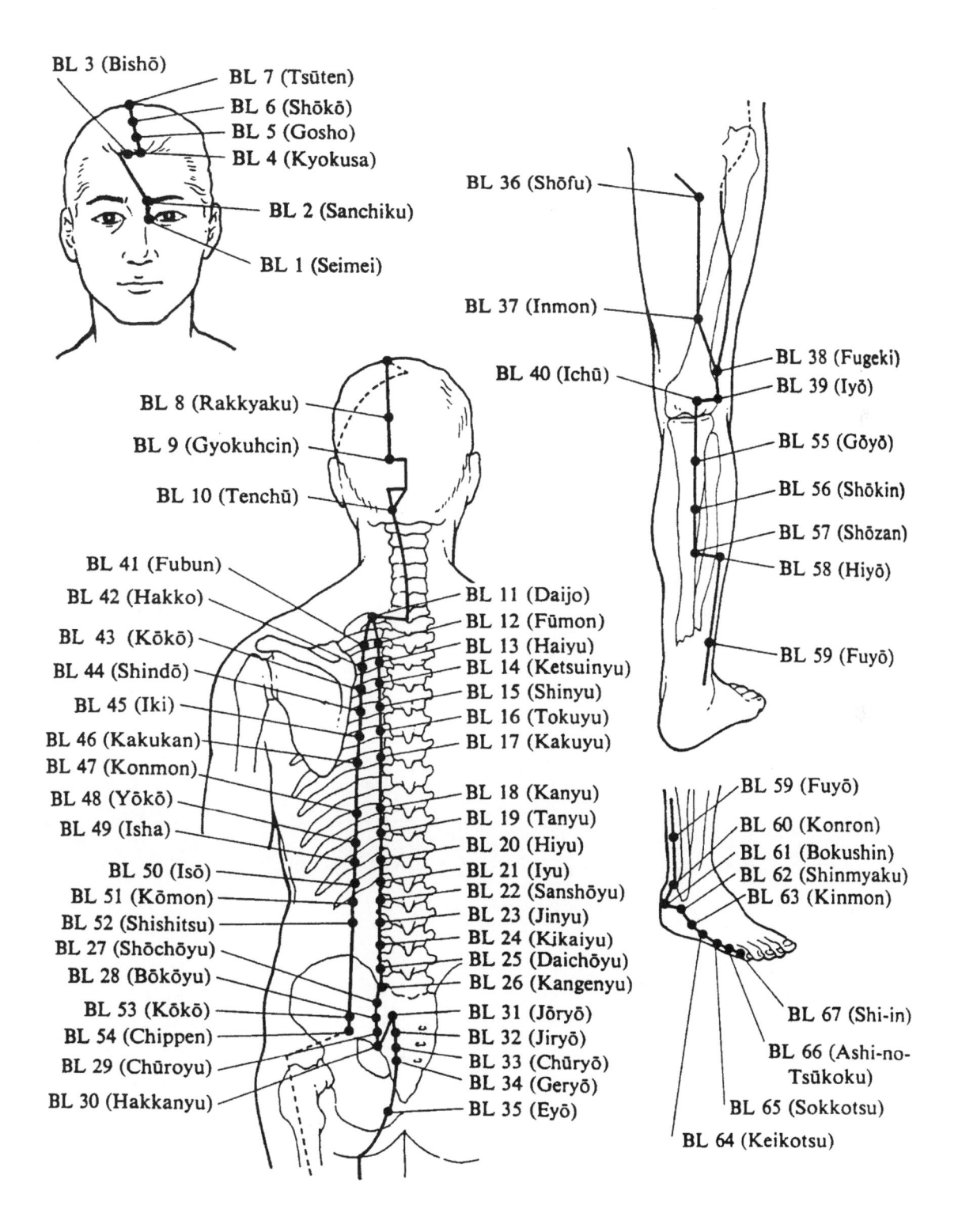

BL 3 (Bishō)
BL 7 (Tsūten)
BL 6 (Shōkō)
BL 5 (Gosho)
BL 4 (Kyokusa)
BL 2 (Sanchiku)
BL 1 (Seimei)

BL 36 (Shōfu)
BL 37 (Inmon)
BL 40 (Ichū)
BL 38 (Fugeki)
BL 39 (Iyō)
BL 55 (Gōyō)
BL 56 (Shōkin)
BL 57 (Shōzan)
BL 58 (Hiyō)
BL 59 (Fuyō)

BL 8 (Rakkyaku)
BL 9 (Gyokuhcin)
BL 10 (Tenchū)

BL 41 (Fubun)
BL 42 (Hakko)
BL 43 (Kōkō)
BL 44 (Shindō)
BL 45 (Iki)
BL 46 (Kakukan)
BL 47 (Konmon)
BL 48 (Yōkō)
BL 49 (Isha)
BL 50 (Isō)
BL 51 (Kōmon)
BL 52 (Shishitsu)
BL 27 (Shōchōyu)
BL 28 (Bōkōyu)
BL 53 (Kōkō)
BL 54 (Chippen)
BL 29 (Chūroyu)
BL 30 (Hakkanyu)

BL 11 (Daijo)
BL 12 (Fūmon)
BL 13 (Haiyu)
BL 14 (Ketsuinyu)
BL 15 (Shinyu)
BL 16 (Tokuyu)
BL 17 (Kakuyu)
BL 18 (Kanyu)
BL 19 (Tanyu)
BL 20 (Hiyu)
BL 21 (Iyu)
BL 22 (Sanshōyu)
BL 23 (Jinyu)
BL 24 (Kikaiyu)
BL 25 (Daichōyu)
BL 26 (Kangenyu)
BL 31 (Jōryō)
BL 32 (Jiryō)
BL 33 (Chūryō)
BL 34 (Geryō)
BL 35 (Eyō)

BL 59 (Fuyō)
BL 60 (Konron)
BL 61 (Bokushin)
BL 62 (Shinmyaku)
BL 63 (Kinmon)
BL 67 (Shi-in)
BL 66 (Ashi-no-Tsūkoku)
BL 65 (Sokkotsu)
BL 64 (Keikotsu)

Active 3-5 pm

LIVER

The Liver corresponds to the wood phase, the direction east, the spring season, the climatic condition of wind, the color of green, the emotion of anger, the sour taste, the goatish odor, and the sound of shouting. Their point of entry is the eyes. They control the sinews (muscles, joints), and their health is reflected in the nails.

The Liver is responsible for spreading and regulating the Qi throughout the body. Its character is flowing and free. Thus, depression or frustration can disturb its function. It is also responsible for storing Blood when the body is at rest. This characteristic, combined with its control over the lower abdomen, makes it the most important Organ with regard to women's menstrual cycle and sexuality.

Depression or long-term frustration can upset the Liver's spreading function and result in continuing depression, a bad temper, and a painful, swollen feeling in the chest and sides. If it worsens, it may lead to disharmony between the Liver and the Stomach and/or Spleen. This disorder is marked by the "rebellion" of Qi in the latter two Organs, whereby the Qi moves in the opposite direction than it is normally proper. In the case of the Stomach, whose Qi normally descends, rebellious Qi means hiccoughing, vomiting, etc. The Qi of the Spleen, on the other hand, is ordinarily directed upward; rebellious Qi in this Organ means diarrhea.

1. The Liver Stores Blood.
One of the Liver's most important functions is storage of Blood, with the emphasis on nourishing and moistening. It regulates the volume of circulating Blood. During activity the Liver will release more Blood for circulation to be sent around the body while during rest, Blood is stored in the Liver. The Liver dominates the Sea of Blood—acupoint Spleen 10, a location that affects blood purity and skin troubles. Deficient Liver Blood:

dry, painful eyes with blurred or weak vision, lack of suppleness or pain in moving the joints, dry skin, dizziness (lack of Blood in the head), and infrequent or spotty menstruation.

2. The Liver Maintains an Unrestricted Condition for Free Flowing Qi.

The Liver makes Qi flow without obstructions both within the Liver and the other Zang-Fu organs. The Liver function is like a tree in spring that grows unobstructed. If restriction occurs so can Rising Liver Fire with symptoms of ill temper, restlessness, headache, vertigo, red face and eyes, and a parched mouth.

3. The Liver Dominates the Tendons.

This also includes the ligaments and finger nails. Deficiency of Liver energy produces under nourishment of the tendons, spasms, numbness, difficulty in contraction, and tremor. If it becomes more serious then it becomes an interior movement of Liver Wind with symptoms of sudden onset of dizziness while moving about, spasms, paralysis, difficulty in movement, or severe vertigo.

4. The Liver Opens into the Eye.

All five pairs of Zang-Fu organs flow through the eye but the Liver, Heart, and Kidney organs have the greater influence.

The Liver Meridian of the Foot (Yin Meridian)

There are 14 points on the Liver meridian. This meridian pertains to the Liver, communicating with the Gall Bladder and connects directly with the Lung, Stomach, and Brain.

Symptoms and Signs

External—Meridian: headache, dizziness, blurred vision, tinnitus (ringing in the ears), fever, spasms of the foot and the hand also may appear in severe cases.

Internal—Organ: fullness and pain in the lower chest, hard lumps in the upper abdomen, abdominal pain, vomiting, jaundice, loose stool, pain in the lower abdomen, hernia, enuresis (bed-wetting), retention of urine, dark urine.

LIVER MERIDIAN

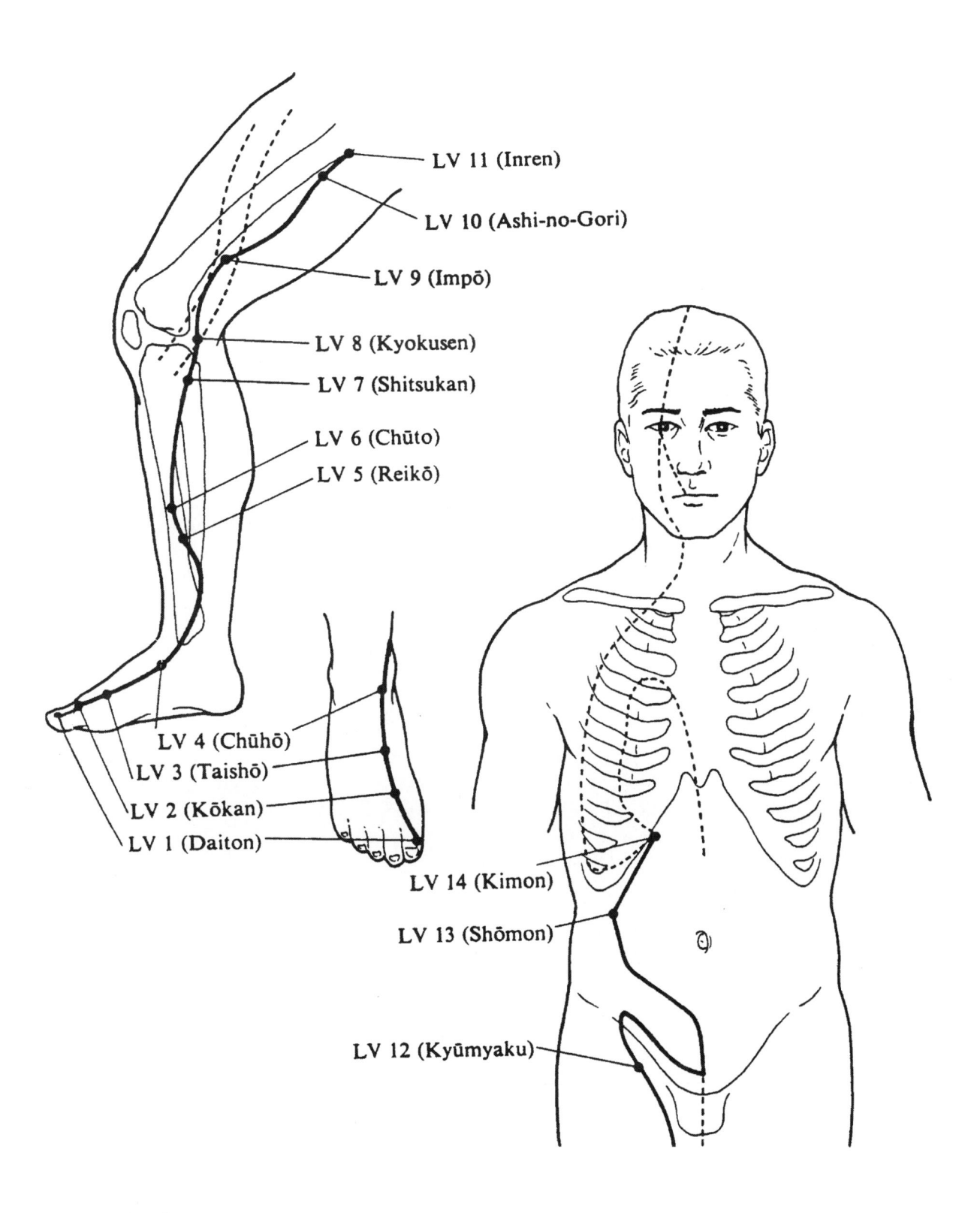

LV 11 (Inren)
LV 10 (Ashi-no-Gori)
LV 9 (Impō)
LV 8 (Kyokusen)
LV 7 (Shitsukan)
LV 6 (Chūto)
LV 5 (Reikō)
LV 4 (Chūhō)
LV 3 (Taishō)
LV 2 (Kōkan)
LV 1 (Daiton)
LV 14 (Kimon)
LV 13 (Shōmon)
LV 12 (Kyūmyaku)

Active 1-3 am

Macrobiotic Shiatsu Workbook

GALL BLADDER

The gall bladder is attached to the lower portion of the liver. Its main function is to store bile produced by the liver and excrete it into the large intestine when fats enter the digestive system. The excretion of bile is controlled by the liver. Problems of the liver will effect the flow of bile. Eating rich foods high in fat such as meats, eggs, oils, and dairy products stimulate bile production. These foods, as well as overeating, promote Damp and Heat to be produced.

For some people bile fluid concentrates and forms stones. If the passage from the gall bladder to the duodenum becomes obstructed or blocked, this usually happens from the presence of cholesterol rich gall stones, the bile goes directly into the blood. This gives the skin a yellowish-green color and the feces become white from lack of bile pigmentation. Other symptoms include an oppressive sensation of fullness in the abdomen and yellow coloring in the eye whites.

The Gall Bladder is sometimes considered an extra Fu organ because food does not actually pass through it. It is also a hollow organ (Fu) but it has a function similar to Zang organs. The Gall Bladder and Liver together are responsible for the movement of unrestrained vital energy.

The Gall Bladder Meridian of the Foot (Yang Meridian)

There are 44 points on this meridian. The Gall Bladder Meridian pertains to the Gall Bladder and communicates with the Liver, and it has some direct connections with the Heart.

Symptoms and Signs

External—Meridian: chill and fever, headache, malaria, gray facial appearance, eye pain, redness in the eyes, pain in the jaw, underarm swelling of lymph nodes (scrofula), pain along the meridian in the hip region, leg, and foot, and deafness.

Internal—Organ: pain in the ribs, vomiting, bitter taste in the mouth, chest pain.

Macrobiotic Shiatsu Workbook

GALL BLADDER MERIDIAN

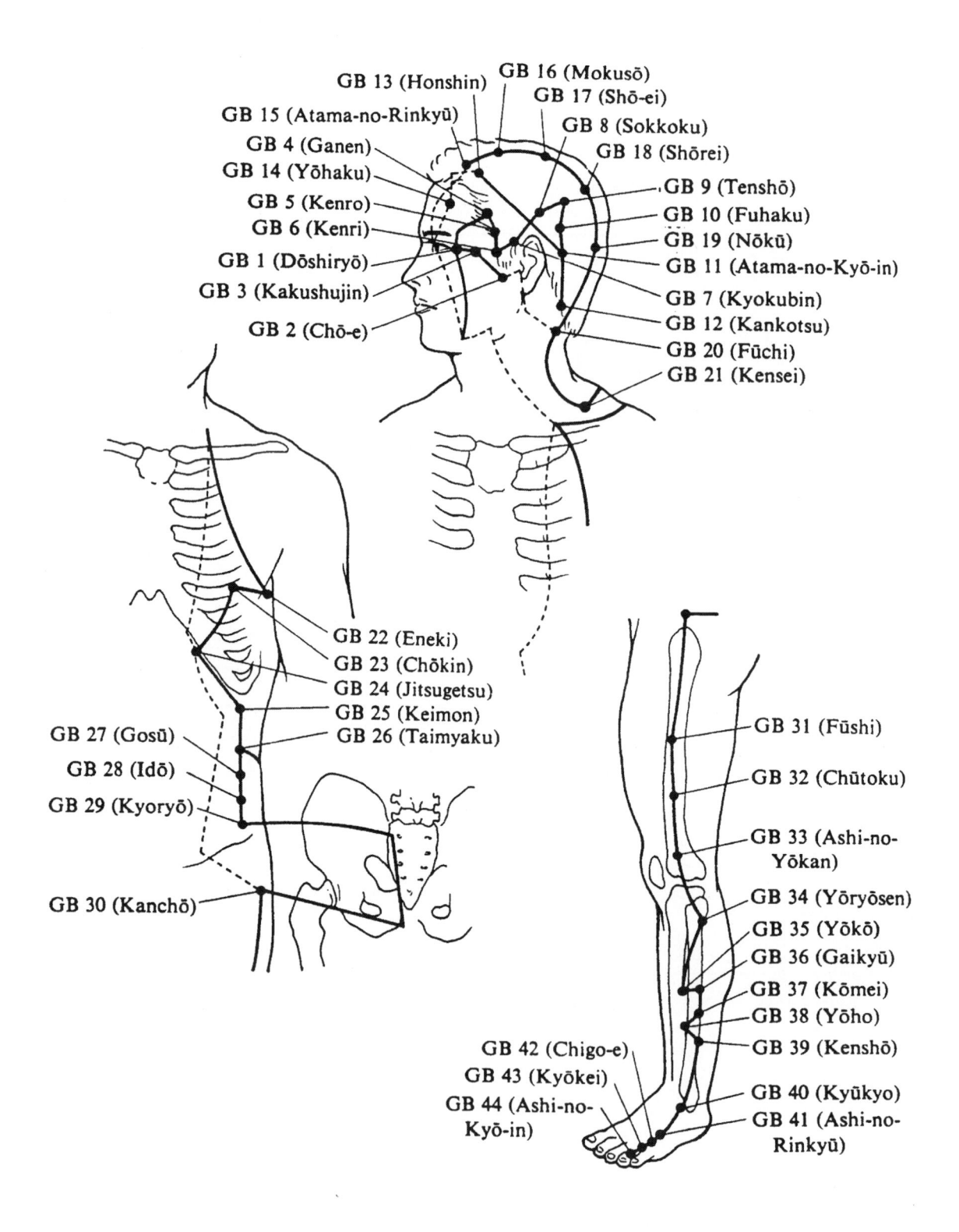

- GB 1 (Dōshiryō)
- GB 2 (Chō-e)
- GB 3 (Kakushujin)
- GB 4 (Ganen)
- GB 5 (Kenro)
- GB 6 (Kenri)
- GB 7 (Kyokubin)
- GB 8 (Sokkoku)
- GB 9 (Tenshō)
- GB 10 (Fuhaku)
- GB 11 (Atama-no-Kyō-in)
- GB 12 (Kankotsu)
- GB 13 (Honshin)
- GB 14 (Yōhaku)
- GB 15 (Atama-no-Rinkyū)
- GB 16 (Mokusō)
- GB 17 (Shō-ei)
- GB 18 (Shōrei)
- GB 19 (Nōkū)
- GB 20 (Fūchi)
- GB 21 (Kensei)
- GB 22 (Eneki)
- GB 23 (Chōkin)
- GB 24 (Jitsugetsu)
- GB 25 (Keimon)
- GB 26 (Taimyaku)
- GB 27 (Gosū)
- GB 28 (Idō)
- GB 29 (Kyoryō)
- GB 30 (Kanchō)
- GB 31 (Fūshi)
- GB 32 (Chūtoku)
- GB 33 (Ashi-no-Yōkan)
- GB 34 (Yōryōsen)
- GB 35 (Yōkō)
- GB 36 (Gaikyū)
- GB 37 (Kōmei)
- GB 38 (Yōho)
- GB 39 (Kenshō)
- GB 40 (Kyūkyo)
- GB 41 (Ashi-no-Rinkyū)
- GB 42 (Chigo-e)
- GB 43 (Kyōkei)
- GB 44 (Ashi-no-Kyō-in)

Active 11 pm -1 am

HEART GOVERNOR (YIN MERIDIAN)

The Heart Governor or Pericardium is considered the outer layer of the heart. The function of the Heart Governor is to protect the Heart from outside disease causing factors. When invasions come it is the Heart Governor that is first affected. The Heart Governor and Triple Heater combined are said to correspond to the "Ministerial Fire" while the Heart and Small Intestine are considered "Sovereign Fire." One common problem of Heart Governor energy is the difficulty in the Heart housing the mind. When this occurs there is loss of consciousness and delirium.

The Heart Governor Meridian of the Hand (Yin Meridian)

There are 9 points on the Heart Governor meridian. The Heart Governor Meridian pertains to the Heart Governor and connects with the Triple Heater, communicating with the Heart and Lung channels.

Symptoms and Signs

External—Meridian: stiff neck, spasms in the arm or leg, flushed face, pain in the eyes, underarm swelling, and hot palms.

Internal— Organs: impaired speech, fainting, irritability, fullness in the chest, palpitations, chest pain, immobility of tongue, and mental disorders.

HEART GOVERNOR MERIDIAN

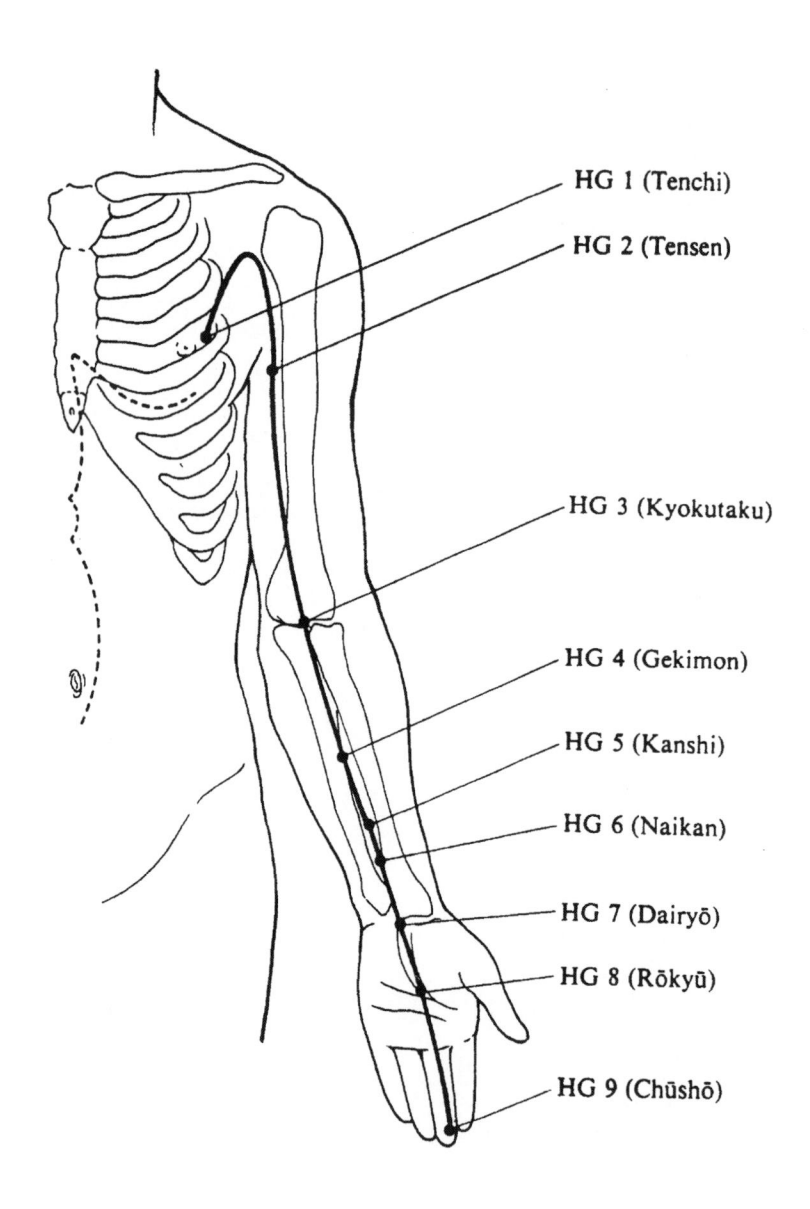

- HG 1 (Tenchi)
- HG 2 (Tensen)
- HG 3 (Kyokutaku)
- HG 4 (Gekimon)
- HG 5 (Kanshi)
- HG 6 (Naikan)
- HG 7 (Dairyō)
- HG 8 (Rōkyū)
- HG 9 (Chūshō)

Active 7-9 pm

TRIPLE HEATER (Sanjiao) (YANG MERIDIAN)

The Triple Heater was described as "having a name but no form" in a third century classic. It is regarded as the function that coordinates all the functions of water metabolism. Its responsibility is to govern all the internal organs in their function to separate the useful from the waste. It also provides water passage for water metabolism. At various times in written literature the "three burners or spaces" were but three regions of the body that were used to group the Organs. The Upper Heater extends from the pharynx to diaphragm and includes the chest, neck, head, and the functions of the Heart and Lungs. The Middle Heater spans the region between the chest and the navel, and includes the functions of the Stomach and Spleen. The Lower Heater contains the lower abdomen and the functions of the Kidneys, Bladder, Large and Small Intestines (and usually the Liver which, however, is sometimes placed in the Middle Heater). As such, the Upper portion has been compared to a mist that spreads the Blood and Qi, the Middle Heater is like a foam that churns up food in the process of digestion, and the Lower Heater is likened to a swamp where all the impure substances are excreted. This description can be used in diagnosis. Symptoms associated with poor function include swelling (edema), bed-wetting (enuresis), excessive urination, and water trapped in the chest (pleural infusion).

The Triple Heater Meridian of the Hand (Yang Meridian)

There are 23 points on the Triple Heater meridian. The Triple Heater Meridian pertains to the Triple Heater and connects with the Heart Governor.

Symptoms and Signs
External—Meridian: swelling and pain in the throat, pain in the cheek and jaw, redness

in the eyes, deafness, pain behind the ear or along the outside of the shoulder and upper arm.

Internal— Organs: abdominal distension, hardness and fullness in the lower abdomen, bed-wetting (enuresis), frequent or excessive urination, painful or impaired passing of urine (dysuria) and edema.

Macrobiotic Shiatsu Workbook

TRIPLE HEATER (SANJIAO) MERIDIAN

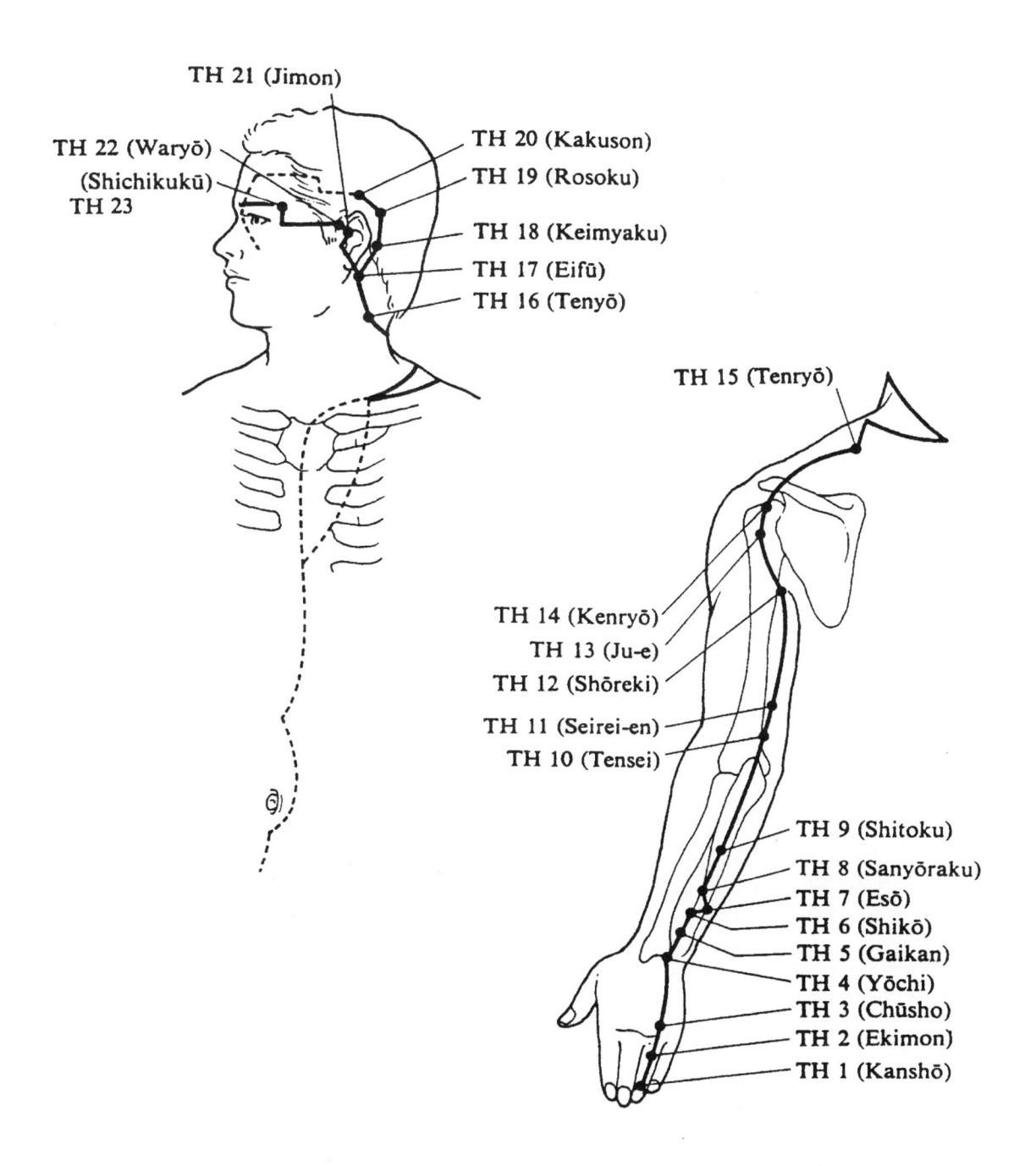

- TH 21 (Jimon)
- TH 22 (Waryō)
- (Shichikukū) TH 23
- TH 20 (Kakuson)
- TH 19 (Rosoku)
- TH 18 (Keimyaku)
- TH 17 (Eifū)
- TH 16 (Tenyō)
- TH 15 (Tenryō)
- TH 14 (Kenryō)
- TH 13 (Ju-e)
- TH 12 (Shōreki)
- TH 11 (Seirei-en)
- TH 10 (Tensei)
- TH 9 (Shitoku)
- TH 8 (Sanyōraku)
- TH 7 (Esō)
- TH 6 (Shikō)
- TH 5 (Gaikan)
- TH 4 (Yōchi)
- TH 3 (Chūsho)
- TH 2 (Ekimon)
- TH 1 (Kanshō)

Active 9-11 pm

77

GOVERNING VESSEL (YANG MERIDIAN)

The Governing Vessel flows from the anus area up the center of the back over the neck and head to inside the upper lip. There are 28 points on this meridian. This regulates all the Yang meridians. *(First name next to acupoint number is Japanese, second name is Chinese)*

Symptoms and Signs

Tetanus, shaking, convulsion, apoplexy (stroke), aphasia (inability to speak after stroke), epilepsy, headache, redness and swelling of the eye, excessive tearing, lumbago, pain in the leg, knee and the back, febrile disease, sore throat, toothache, swelling in the gums, numbness of foot and hand, and night sweating.

The Governing Vessel acupoints located on the head and the neck, are usually indicated for disorders of head, brain, and febrile diseases. The points on the back are indicated for the diseases of the lung, the heart, the pericardium, the liver, gall bladder, spleen, stomach, and diseases of the back, loin, and lower extremities while those on the lumbo-sacral region are indicated for diseases of the kidney, bladder, and large and small intestine.

Macrobiotic Shiatsu Workbook

GOVERNING VESSEL MERIDIAN

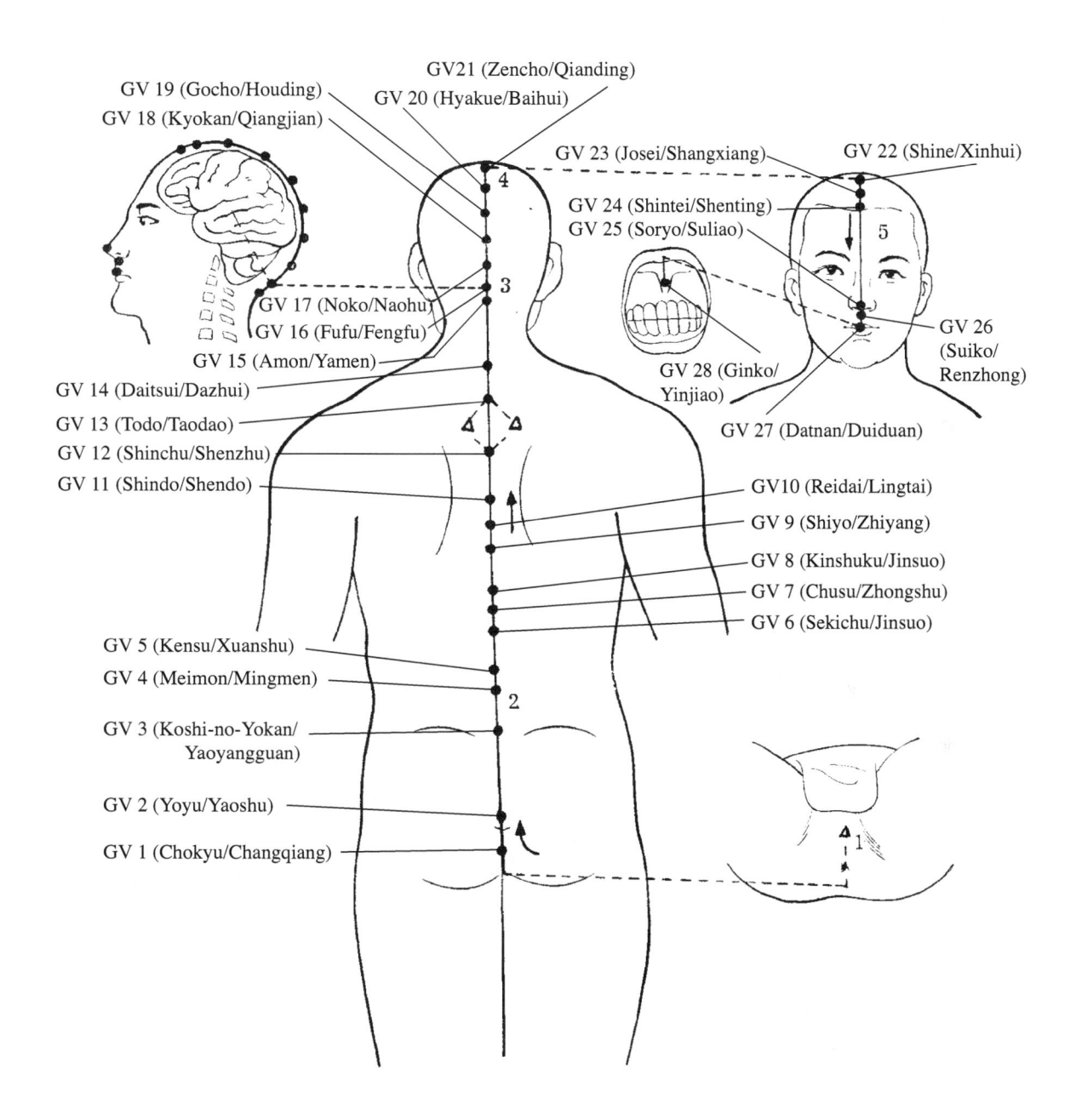

- GV 1 (Chokyu/Changqiang)
- GV 2 (Yoyu/Yaoshu)
- GV 3 (Koshi-no-Yokan/Yaoyangguan)
- GV 4 (Meimon/Mingmen)
- GV 5 (Kensu/Xuanshu)
- GV 6 (Sekichu/Jinsuo)
- GV 7 (Chusu/Zhongshu)
- GV 8 (Kinshuku/Jinsuo)
- GV 9 (Shiyo/Zhiyang)
- GV 10 (Reidai/Lingtai)
- GV 11 (Shindo/Shendo)
- GV 12 (Shinchu/Shenzhu)
- GV 13 (Todo/Taodao)
- GV 14 (Daitsui/Dazhui)
- GV 15 (Amon/Yamen)
- GV 16 (Fufu/Fengfu)
- GV 17 (Noko/Naohu)
- GV 18 (Kyokan/Qiangjian)
- GV 19 (Gocho/Houding)
- GV 20 (Hyakue/Baihui)
- GV 21 (Zencho/Qianding)
- GV 22 (Shine/Xinhui)
- GV 23 (Josei/Shangxiang)
- GV 24 (Shintei/Shenting)
- GV 25 (Soryo/Suliao)
- GV 26 (Suiko/Renzhong)
- GV 27 (Datnan/Duiduan)
- GV 28 (Ginko/Yinjiao)

79

CONCEPTION VESSEL (YIN MERIDIAN)

There are 24 points on this meridian. It regulates the functions of all Yin meridians and nourishes the fetus. Its function is closely related with pregnancy and therefore has intimate links with the Kidneys and uterus. *(First name next to acupoint number is Japanese, second name is Chinese)*

Symptoms and Signs

Hemorrhoids, diarrhea, dysentery, malaria, cough, hemoptysis (coughing up blood), toothache, swelling of pharynx, dysuria (painful urination), pain in the abdomen, difficulty swallowing, post obstetrical palsy, lumbago, cold sensation in the umbilical region, vomiting, hiccup, and pain in the breast. It also affects the throat, chest abdomen, umbilical region, diseases of the digestive and urogenital systems, and cold diseases.

CONCEPTION VESSEL MERIDIAN

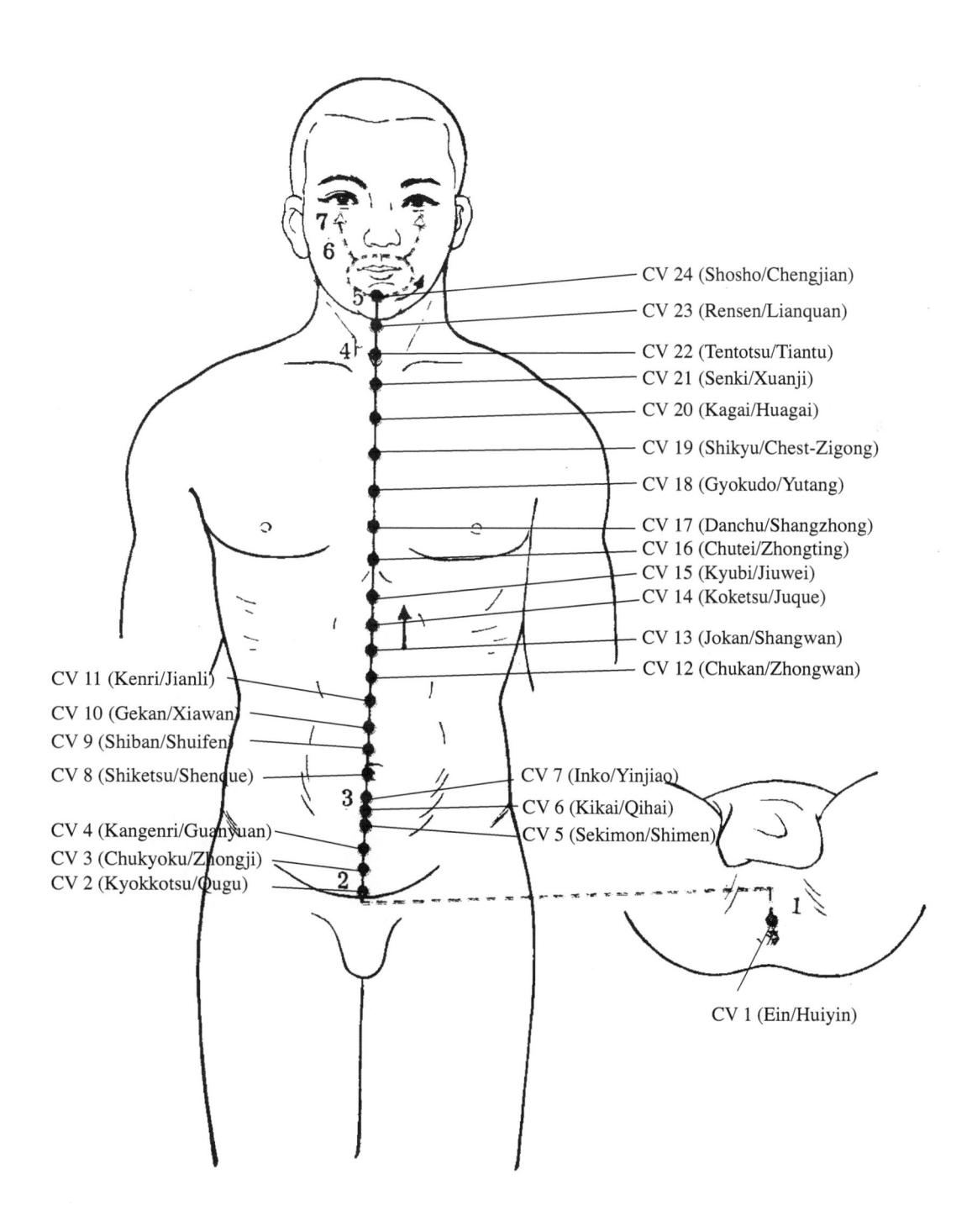

- CV 24 (Shosho/Chengjian)
- CV 23 (Rensen/Lianquan)
- CV 22 (Tentotsu/Tiantu)
- CV 21 (Senki/Xuanji)
- CV 20 (Kagai/Huagai)
- CV 19 (Shikyu/Chest-Zigong)
- CV 18 (Gyokudo/Yutang)
- CV 17 (Danchu/Shangzhong)
- CV 16 (Chutei/Zhongting)
- CV 15 (Kyubi/Jiuwei)
- CV 14 (Koketsu/Juque)
- CV 13 (Jokan/Shangwan)
- CV 12 (Chukan/Zhongwan)
- CV 11 (Kenri/Jianli)
- CV 10 (Gekan/Xiawan)
- CV 9 (Shiban/Shuifen)
- CV 8 (Shiketsu/Shenque)
- CV 7 (Inko/Yinjiao)
- CV 6 (Kikai/Qihai)
- CV 5 (Sekimon/Shimen)
- CV 4 (Kangenri/Guanyuan)
- CV 3 (Chukyoku/Zhongji)
- CV 2 (Kyokkotsu/Qugu)
- CV 1 (Ein/Huiyin)

Summary of Meridian Pathology

The Three Arm Yin Meridians

    1. Arm Greater Yin **Lung** meridian is indicated for diseases of the chest, throat, trachea, nose and Lung.

    2. Arm Absolute Yin **Heart Governor** meridian is indicated for diseases of the chest, Stomach, and Heart, as well as mental disorder generally.

    3. Arm Lesser Yin **Heart** meridian is indicated for diseases of the chest, tongue and Heart, as well as mental disorders generally.

The Three Arm Yang Meridians

    1. Arm Yang Brightness **Large Intestine** meridian is indicated for diseases of the face, eyes, ears, nose, gums, throat and Large Intestine, as well as febrile diseases generally.

    2. Arm Lesser Yang **Triple Heater** meridian is indicated for diseases of the temporal region, eyes, ears, throat and ribs, as well as febrile diseases generally.

    3. Arm Greater Yang **Small Intestine** meridian is indicated for diseases of the eyes, ears, throat, as well as mental disorders generally.

The Three Leg Yang Meridians

    1. Leg Yang Brightness **Stomach** meridian is indicated for diseases of the face, nose, gums, throat, Stomach and Intestines as well as mental and febrile diseases generally.

    2. Leg Lesser Yang **Gall Bladder** meridian is indicated or diseases of the temporal region, nose, eyes, throat and ribs, as well as febrile diseases generally.

3\. Leg Greater Yang **Bladder** meridian is indicated for diseases affecting the nose, eyes and lumbar region, as well as febrile and mental diseases generally.

The Three Leg Yin Meridians

1\. Leg Greater Yin **Spleen** meridian is indicated for diseases of the upper abdomen, Stomach, Intestines, and Urogenital system.

2\. Leg Absolute Yin **Liver** meridian is indicated for diseases affecting the hypochondriac region, lower abdomen, urogenital system and head.

3\. Leg Lesser Yin **Kidney** meridian is indicated for diseases affecting the waist, urogenital system, throat and mental disorders generally.

Circulating Direction of the Meridians

Downward Movement	Upward Movement
Lungs	Large Intestine
Heart	Small Intestine
Heart Governor	Triple Heater
Stomach	Spleen
Bladder	Kidney
Gall Bladder	Liver

Natural Home Remedies Index

Brown Rice Cream 85	Salt Pack 92
Pearl Barley (semen coix) 85	Salt Water Wash 93
Miso Soup 85	Bancha (Kukicha) Douche 93
Shredded Kombu Soup 86	Kombu Water 93
Carp Soup (Koi Koku) 86	Hijiki-Vegetable Sauté 93
Aduki/Kombu/Squash 87	Nori Condiment 94
Carrot/Daikon Mixture 87	Shio Kombu 94
Umeboshi 87	Roasted Sea Vegetable Powder 94
Baked Umeboshi or Ume Pits 87	Seaweed Powder w/Seeds 95
Shiitake Mushroom 88	Brown Rice Tea 95
Black Soy Beans 88	Barley Tea 96
Gomasio (Sesame Salt) 88	Barley/Aduki Tea 96
Tekka 89	Aduki Bean Tea 96
Shiso 89	Kombu Tea 96
Small Dried Fish (Chirimen) 89	Sweet Vegetable Drink 97
Rice or Barley/Greens Plaster 89	Daikon Drink No. 1 97
Buckwheat Plaster 90	Daikon Drink No. 2 97
Green Plaster 90	Lotus Tea 97
Miso Plaster 90	Kombu/Shiitake Broth 98
Taro Plaster 90	Shiitake Tea 98
Potato Plaster 91	Ume Concentrate 98
Ginger Compress 91	Reishi Tea 98
Ginger Oil 91	Ume/Sho/Bancha Drink 99
Sesame Oil 92	Umeboshi Kuzu Drink 99
Body Scrub 92	Ame Kuzu Drink 99
Salt Bath 92	

Natural Home Remedies

BROWN RICE CREAM

In a cask iron skillet dry roast 1 cup of brown rice until it is golden color. Do not use oil. Put rice in a pot, add 7-10 cups of purified water (not chlorinated tap water) and bring to a boil. Cover, lower the flame and simmer 3-4 hours. It is quicker to use a pressure cooker. Reduce water to 5 cups and pressure cook for 2 hours. Squeeze cooled contents through a cotton cheese cloth (or a Foley food mill) and save. Add sea salt to your portion as you use it. It can be eaten as is or topped with sesame salt or nori.

Uses: recovering from sickness, fatigue, and lack of appetite.

PEARL BARLEY (SEMEN COIX)

Make a soup using 1 cup cooked Pearl Barley, carrots, onions, wakame sea vegetable and enough water to make soup consistency. Season to taste. Eat 1 bowl per day. Another method of using pearl barley is to add 10 percent pearl barley to brown rice. Eat regularly.

Uses: hemorrhoids, warts, moles, some cancers, and the side effects of chemotherapy and radiation. Pearl barley, known as Job's Tears and Hato Mugi in Japanese has been used to reduce tumors, swelling, inflammation, and heat in the body.

MISO SOUP
4 cups water
6 inch piece wakame sea vegetable
1/4 cup each of onion, carrot, green vegetable or wild greens
1/2 inch slice tofu (cubed)
1/4 cup barley (or brown rice or hatcho) miso

Place sea vegetable and water in soup pot and bring to boil. Simmer while cut the vegetables to similar size and shape. Remove sea vegetable, cool briefly and cut. Return chopped sea vegetable to pot. Add all ingredients to soup pot except miso and slow boil until done, up to one-half hour, depending on how vegetables are cut. Soup vegetables are well cooked so they melt in our mouth. A side dish of vegetables may be more lightly cooked. Dilute miso in a little of the hot soup liquid and add during the last three minutes of gentle simmering. It's important not to cook the miso at a rolling boil that would kill the beneficial bacteria. Use organic ingredients, 1-3 year old, unpasteurized miso.

Uses: for strength, stamina, supports metabolism, prevents allergies, and increases circulation, purifies blood.

SHREDDED KOMBU SOUP

Add 1-2 tablespoons of shredded kombu to miso soup. Or add to hot water, stir, season with shoyu (soy sauce) and eat.

Uses: for fatigue, cleans the blood.

CARP SOUP (KOI KOKU)
1 pound fresh carp (trout or snapper can be use instead)
1-1 1/2 pound burdock root
1 tablespoon oil
3/4 cup barley miso
1/4 cup used bancha leaves
1/4 teaspoon fresh grated ginger

Cut fish into 1 inch pieces. Cut burdock into thinly shaved pieces, like sharpening a pencil with a knife. Saute the burdock for 10-20 minutes in oil. Add the fish and cover with enough water to cover over fish with 2 inches. Tie some bancha or Kukicha leftovers together in a cheesecloth. Add this sack to soup pot. The tea leaves or twigs will help soften the fish bones. Bring to a boil and cook for at least 2 hours (up to 4-8 hours) on a low flame. If you use a pressure cooker cook for 1-2 hours. Remove the tea bag and add miso and ginger. Season to taste. Simmer for 10 minutes. Garnish with chopped scallions. Eat 1-2 bowls per day. Variation: instead of carp with burdock, you can use snapper or trout with carrots.

Uses: strengthens the whole system, decreased energy, decreased sexual vitality, lack of mother's milk, and anemia.

ADUKI/KOMBU/SQUASH
1 cup aduki beans
2 cups squash
2 six inch pieces of kombu sea vegetable

Wash aduki beans. Cut soaked kombu sea vegetable into 1 inch pieces. Place kombu pieces in the bottom of a pot, and place aduki beans on top. Cover with water. Bring to a boil and simmer for 40 minutes. Add squash. Sprinkle with sea salt. Cover and cook for 30 minutes more. Be sure enough water is in pot. Season to taste with sea salt or tamari.

Uses: helpful in regulating the blood sugar level such as hypoglycemia and diabetes, useful in taming the sweet craving, lack of vitality, good for any kidney problem. Some people enjoy it as a dessert.

CARROT/DAIKON MIXTURE
1/4 cup grated daikon
1/4 cup grated carrot
1/4 teaspoon fresh grated ginger
1/2 ume or 1/2 teaspoon paste

Pour 1/2 cup twig tea over ingredients, add 1 teaspoon green nori flakes. Take on empty stomach before breakfast. Wait 30-60 minutes before eating.

Uses: breaks up accumulated fat. Good for over-weight people to skip breakfast, this way they will lose weight quickly.

UMEBOSHI

Cook 1 umeboshi with brown rice instead of using sea salt.

Add umeboshi pieces to center of brown rice balls to be used a snack or travel food.

Eat as is. Add umeboshi pieces to hot water or tea.

Uses: a powerful and useful food, good for food poisoning, upset stomach, water contamination, diarrhea, constipation, motion sickness, headache, and decreases fatigue.

BAKED UMEBOSHI or UMEBOSHI PITS

Roast the plum or saved pits in the oven at a very high temperature. Crush them into a black powder. Store in sealed container. Use 1/2 -1 teaspoon charred powder mixed with 1 cup water or tea. If you crush the pit you will find a seed inside. Eat this seed it contains vitamin B17 (laetrile)—an anticancer agent. Bake umeboshi is a very yang preparation.

Uses: getting rid of unfriendly intestinal bacteria, painful gas buildup, intestinal cancer, stomach ulcer, colds, and diarrhea. Good for strengthening the immune system.

SHIITAKE MUSHROOM

Cook with other vegetables or add to soup. Dried shiitake, reconstituted with water and cooked can be used 2-3 times per week.

Uses: good source of protein, contains anticancer agents, breaks up fat, eliminates cholesterol, and relaxes an over tense or stressed body. It is not a good idea to eat any variety of mushroom raw.

BLACK SOY BEANS

Soak overnight and cook 10 percent black soy beans in with brown rice. Eat 2-3 times per week. Can also be used in a soup. Can also be used as a tea.

Uses: good for constipation, female troubles such as menstruation irregularities, and hardening or swelling of the breast.

GOMASIO (SESAME SALT CONDIMENT)

Roast 1-3 teaspoons unrefined sea salt in skillet until dry, about 1-2 minutes. Place roasted salt in mortar or suribachi. Add 1 cup whole (unhulled) sesame seeds in the skillet and stir over medium heat until they taste good, are dry, or crush easily between the pressure of 2 fingers, 5-10 minutes. If seeds pop a lot, heat is too high. Grind salt, then add seeds and grind together until half the seeds are pulverized, about 5-10 minutes. Store in a sealed container. Use 1/4-1/2 teaspoon on grains and vegetables.

Uses: stimulates the appetite and tastes good, good for over acidity, relieves tiredness, strengthens the nervous system.

TEKKA

Tekka is a mixture of burdock root, carrot, lotus root, grated ginger, miso, and sesame oil roasted together for a long time in a cast iron skillet. Buy prepared Tekka seasoning at natural foods stores, use 1/4-1/2 teaspoon on grains and vegetables.

Uses: fatigue, anemia, as a tonic, influences asthma, diarrhea, strengthens the heart.

SHISO

Shiso is the purple/red leaf the comes in umeboshi and that gives the ume its distinctive color and flavor. The leaf is high in calcium, iron, and vitamins A, B2, C. Use as sprinkling on grains and vegetables.

Uses: anemia, cough, lack of urine production, irritability, common colds.

SMALL DRIED FISH (CHIRIMEN)

Sprinkle small portion of ground up chirimen (very small dried sardine-like fish obtained from Asian markets) on grains. You also can soak in water until soft, 15-30 minutes, and add to moist wakame sea vegetable. Season with brown rice vinegar and soy sauce for salad.

Uses: good for poor digestion, osteoporosis, lack of calcium, mineral and protein source.

BROWN RICE or BARLEY/GREENS PLASTER

Mix 70 percent cooked grain with 30 percent raw green leaves in a mortar and pestle or suribachi. Add 1/2 teaspoon of fresh grated ginger. Crush this mixture together. Spread on cotton towel approximately 1/2 inch thick and place on body area to be treated. The grain/green mixture touches the skin directly. Secure in place for 4 hours or overnight. Continue until you feel better.

Uses: to reduce swelling and inflammation, pain, and itch. Good on boils, sore spots, insect bites, lymph nodes, breast, and bruises

BUCKWHEAT PLASTER

Mix buckwheat flour with enough warm water and knead it to obtain a stiff dough that is not too wet. Spread 3/4 inch layer directly on the skin, and hold it in place with a piece of cotton cloth. Remove after 1-2 hours, or when the dough has become soft and watery. Replace the plaster with a fresh one. Must be applied often to get results.

Uses: to remove excess water, can be used on the abdomen, pleural cavity, or on joints, can be applied on the bladder area to increase possibility of urinating.

GREEN PLASTER

Mash up 2-3 leaves of cabbage greens or other available green leafy vegetable, and place directly on affected area. When leaves are warm, replace with fresh compress.

Uses: to draw heat out of the body, inflammatory conditions such as mumps.

MISO PLASTER

In a sauce pan, heat up miso mixed with water to consistency like cottage cheese. Pour liquid onto towel and place on area you want to treat such as the abdomen. Cover with a dry towel to retain heat longer. Warm again when cool.

Uses: for any cold conditions and swollen abdomen.

TARO PLASTER

Wash 3-4 taro potato roots and peel off the skins. Grate the remaining potatoes and add enough white flour to bind the mash. You do not want the mixture to be too dry. If it is too dry it will lose its drawing power. Add 1 teaspoon of fresh grated ginger root. Spread mixture on a damp cotton towel or cheesecloth about 1/2 inch thick. Place plaster on affected area so that the taro mixture is directly on the skin. Secure and keep on for 2-4 hours.

Uses: cooling agent to reduce heat or inflammation, reduces trauma induced swelling and pain, helpful in reducing hardness and size of some tumors.

POTATO PLASTER

Peel and grate regular potatoes. This makes a moist paste. Mix with enough white flour to make it stick together. Add 1 teaspoon of fresh grated ginger root. Spread mixture on a damp cotton towel or cheesecloth about 1/2 inch thick. Place plaster on affected area so that the potato mixture is directly on the skin. Secure and keep on for 2-4 hours.

Uses: cooling agent to reduce heat or inflammation, reduces trauma induced swelling and pain, helpful in reducing hardness and size of some tumors. This plaster is less strong then taro potato plasters.

GINGER COMPRESS

Bring 3-4 quarts of water to boil, place about a golf ball size of fresh grated ginger root in a cotton cloth, cheesecloth, or a handkerchief. Put this ball into the boiled water that is now just below the boiling point. Don't let the liquid boil again as this lessens it effectiveness. The mixture is now ready to use. Dip a towel into the hot ginger water trying to keep the ends dry, as the liquid is very hot. Hold by the ends of the towel and dip in the center portion., Wring it out and place directly on the area to be treated. Place a second, dry towel on top to reduce heat loss. Apply a fresh hot towel every minute or so and continue until the skin becomes red, about 15-20 minutes.

Uses: muscle tension, promotes circulation of body fluids such as blood and lymph fluid, it has a stimulating effect, reduces stagnation, used for 3-5 minutes before a Taro Plaster to warm area.

GINGER OIL

Mix 1 part pure sesame oil and 1 part fresh squeezed ginger juice together. Grated ginger on a cheese grater. Store in refrigerator. Use small amount rubbed and skin and/or spine.

Uses: increase skin circulation, warms body, stimulates spine and nervous system.

SESAME OIL

Sesame oil is my favorite oil. Toasted sesame oil is tasty. For variety use regular, toasted, and dark toasted sesame oil.

Uses: good for burns, after soaking minor burn area in cool salted water; good for dry skin, cracked nipples; in the eye—first boil the oil, then strain it through sterile gauze. With an eye dropper, put 2-3 drops in eye before sleep. It stings then pushes excess water out of the eye.

BODY SCRUB

Dip a small cotton towel or cloth in hot water. Wring out the excess water. Scrub the whole body, dipping the towel into hot water again when cool. Be sure to include the hands and feet and each finger and toe. The skin should become pink or slightly red.

Uses: activates circulation and better energy flow through the entire body. It helps to discharge fat accumulated under the skin and opens pores to promote smooth and regular elimination of toxins.

SALT BATH

Add 3 cups of sea salt to normal sized bath. Add very warm to hot water. Sit and relax for 10-20 minutes.

Uses: relaxes and over tense body; increases circulation, especially lower portions; draws toxins out of the body.

SALT PACK

Roast 1-11/2 cups sea salt in a dry pan until hot and then wrap in a thick cotton linen or towel. Apply to the troubled area. Change when the pack begins to cool.

Uses: abdominal cramps, menstrual cramps, diarrhea, ear pain such as after swimming, can be used to warm cool areas.

SALT WATER WASH

Dissolve small amount of sea salt in pure water. Taste should be salty like the ocean.

Uses: for inflamed or sore throat, gargle with mixture; for nasal obstruction and tendency toward excess mucus production and nasal trouble, rinse the sinuses by sniffing salt water up the nostrils; for eye redness, burning, allergy reactions, wash eyes with solution by placing water in an eye cup, placing over one opened eye for 3-5 seconds. Repeat with other eye.

BANCHA (KUKICHA) DOUCHE

Use one quart bancha (kukicha/twig) tea, cooled to body temperature. Add one three-finger pinch of sea salt plus one teaspoon of brown rice vinegar. Stir all together, pour into douche bag, and douche after a Daikon Hip or Salt Water Bath.

Uses: helps to eliminate stagnated mucus and fat in the region of the uterus and vagina.

KOMBU WATER

Place 1 piece of kombu sea vegetable in 2 quarts of water to soak overnight. Use water for everything from soups and teas, to steaming broth and water for your plants.

Uses: all sea vegetables are effective in dealing with environmental pollutants including radiation. They are also good sources of iodine and positively affect the thyroid gland.

HIJIKI-VEGETABLE SAUTÉ
1/2 cup hijiki sea vegetable
2 cups water
1 teaspoon- 1 tablespoon sesame oil (optional)
1 cup onion, thinly sliced
1 cup carrot, thinly sliced in matchsticks
2 tablespoons natural soy sauce
2 tablespoons parsley or green onion tops

Soak hijiki in water until reconstituted, about 20 minutes. In a large skillet, heat oil and sauté onion and carrot briefly. Push vegetables to side of pan, and transfer hijiki to pan. Put vegetables on top of hijiki. Pour soak water over hijiki to a depth of 1/2 inch. Take care to avoid using the last bit of water where sand or other particles may have settled. Cover and bring to boil, then turn heat to medium-low to slow-boil until done, about 15 minutes. Broth should be evaporated. Add soy sauce and parsley or green onion tops and cook a couple of minutes more, uncovered. You can substitute arame for hijiki.

Use: good for osteoporosis and other bone illnesses because of high calcium content, anemia, high blood pressure, allergies, arthritis, rheumatism, and nervous disorders.

NORI CONDIMENT

Tear up 3-4 sheets of toasted nori sea vegetable into a frying pan. Add a little water and tamari to moisten. Cook until smooth, approximately 15 minutes so that very little liquid remains and you are left with a paste. Eat 1 teaspoon per day on rice.

Uses: good for lack of strength, fatigue, lack of appetite. It cleans the blood by supplying minerals.

SHIO KOMBU

Start with left over kombu from soaking. Chop into 1 inch squares. Cover with a 50/50 mixture of water and tamari. Heat until soft. Be sure enough liquid is present to prevent burning. When it is ready all liquid should be allow to evaporate. Use 1-2 pieces per meal.

Uses: fatigue, mentally weak or dull, lack of concentration, strengthens the immune system.

ROASTED SEA VEGETABLE POWDER

Place whole package of sea vegetable on cookie sheet in preheated 350 degree oven. Bake for 3-5 minutes for most sea vegetables, or up to 10-15 minutes for wakame. Over cooking makes it taste bitter. Pulverize into powder with your hands or a mortar and pestle (or suribachi). Two cups dry seaweed, baked and pulverized, yields just 1/2 cup flakes or 2 tablespoons powder. Store in tightly covered container. Use in soups or on grains and vegetables.

Uses: good for fatigue, helpful in chronic fatigue syndrome, excellent source of minerals the body can assimilate, and helps to stop bleeding.

ROASTED SEAWEED POWDER WITH SEEDS
2 cups dry dulse, wild nori, or wakame or 1/4 cup packaged nori or dulse flakes
1 cup seeds (sunflower, pumpkin, or sesame)
1/2-1 tablespoon natural soy sauce

Bake sea vegetable on cookie sheet in preheated 350 degree oven. Bake for 3-5 minutes for most sea vegetables, or up to 10-15 minutes for wakame. Over cooking makes it taste bitter. Pulverize into powder with your hands or a mortar and pestle (or suribachi). Then bake seeds in same oven for 10-15 minutes, checking seeds after 8 minutes. Sprinkle or spray seeds with soy sauce, stir, and return seeds to over to toast until dry, about 2 minutes more. Instead of baking, a dry skillet may be used on stove-top, but this method demands constant attention. Crush seeds with a rolling pin and mix with crumbled sea vegetables. Store in tightly covered container. Use in soups or on grains and vegetables.

Uses: good for fatigue, helpful in chronic fatigue syndrome, excellent source of minerals the body can assimilate.

BROWN RICE TEA

In a cast iron skillet, dry roast 1/2 cup of washed brown rice. Roast it to a golden yellow color. Place in sauce pan and add 1 quart water. Bring to boil and simmer for 20-30 minutes. Add a pinch of sea salt during the cooking process. Strain and use 1 cup per serving.

Uses: serves as a nutrient source for those with inability to digest well, good for heating the body during winter.

BARLEY TEA

In a cast iron skillet, dry roast 1/2 cup of washed barley. Roast it to a golden brown color. Place in sauce pan and add 1 quart water. Bring to boil and simmer for 20-30 minutes. Add a pinch of sea salt during the cooking process. Strain and use 1 cup per serving.

Uses: serves as a nutrient source for those with inability to digest well, good for cooling the body during summer.

BARLEY/ADUKI TEA

1/4 cup Pearl Barley (hato mugi)
1/4 cup Aduki Beans
1 six inch piece of Kombu sea vegetable
1 quart of water

Mix all ingredients together in sauce pan. Bring to boil and simmer for 30-40 minutes. Strain and use broth.

Uses: increases circulation to the skin, cleanses the kidneys, easy to absorb nutrient source for weak and under weight people, positively affects spleen and lymphatic system.

ADUKI BEAN TEA

Place one cup of beans in a pot with a two-inch strip of kombu (soaked and finely chopped). Add four cups of water and bring to a boil. Lower the flame, cover and simmer for one-half hour. Strain out the beans and drink the liquid while hot.

Uses: helps to regulate the kidney and urinary function. Also good for constipation.

KOMBU TEA

Boil a 6 inch strip of kombu in a quart of water for 15 minutes.

Uses: cleans and strengthens the blood, strengthens and calms the nervous system, positively affects the immune system.

SWEET VEGETABLE DRINK

Dice and mix together 4 kinds of round and sweet vegetables to make 1 cup. Use winter squash, cabbages, carrot, daikon, onion, and kombu. Add assorted 1 cup of vegetables to 1 quart of water. Simmer for 10-15 minutes. Strain and use liquid. Take 1/2-1 cup broth 1-2 times per day.

Uses: maintains constant blood sugar level, helpful for diabetes and hypoglycemia, reduces craving for sweets, positively affects pancreas and spleen.

DAIKON DRINK NO. 1

Grate about 3 tablespoons of fresh daikon. Mix the daikon with one-quarter teaspoon grated ginger and a few drops of soy sauce. Pour two or three cups of hot twig tea over the mixed ingredients. Drink hot. After drinking this tea, go to bed and wrap yourself in a blanket to induce sweating. (Since this tea is strong, do not take more than twice a day for one or two days.)

Uses: lowers fevers by inducing sweating. It brings relief from food poisoning caused by meat, fish, or shellfish.

DAIKON DRINK NO. 2

Grate one-half cup of daikon. Place daikon in a cheesecloth and squeeze out the juice. To two tablespoons of juice, add six tablespoons of water. Bring mixture to a boil and simmer for 30-60 seconds. Add a pinch of sea salt or a few drops of soy sauce. Drink preparation once each day or once every two days, for no more than three times in a row.

Uses: induces urination and relieves swollen ankles and feet.

LOTUS TEA

Grate 2 inch piece of fresh lotus root. Squeeze out its juice through a cheesecloth. Add 2-3 drops of ginger juice and a few grains of sea salt or drops of soy sauce. Add equal volume of water and simmer for a few minutes. Or you can prepare from dried lotus root or lotus root powder. If you use dried lotus root, boil 6-10 slices in 1 cup of water for

15-20 minutes. Add ginger, sea salt and serve. For lotus root powder use 1-2 teaspoons and 1 cup water, simmer for 5 minutes, add ginger juice, sea salt and serve.

Uses: positively affects respiratory system; calms irritated mucus membranes of the lungs; good for bronchitis, asthma, cough; and sinus congestion and infections.

KOMBU/SHIITAKE BROTH

Soak 2-4 shiitake mushrooms and a 6 inch piece of kombu for 30 minutes. Bring to a boil and simmer for 20-30 minutes.

Uses: cleans blood, softens hard condition such as stress, adds minerals to body, can be used as a broth for soups or stews, adds nutrition and flavor.

SHIITAKE TEA

Soak 1-2 dried mushrooms for one hour, or until it is soft. Cut it in quarters, add 2 cups of water, and bring to a boil with a pinch of sea salt. Simmer for about 15-20 minutes, until 1 cup of tea is left. Drink half a cup at a time.

Uses: eliminates the residue of excess protein and salt from the body, relaxes a tense condition, reduces high blood pressure, and increase urine.

UME CONCENTRATE

Mix 1 teaspoon ume concentrate in 1 cup boiled water or twig tea. Stir and drink.

Uses: strengthens and alkalinizes the blood, good for diarrhea, constipation, upset stomach, lack of appetite, headache, and minor food poisoning.

REISHI TEA

Boil 4-8 grams of Reishi mushroom (ganoderma lucidum) with small amount of licorice root in 1 quart of water. Bring to a boil, cover, and simmer for 1 hour. Drink 1/2 - 2 cups, per day.

Uses: general tonic; good for allergies; enhances immune system; positively affects chronic fatigue syndrome; positively affects AIDS (acquired immune deficiency syndrome) and ARC (AIDS related complex); reduces blood pressure; increases circulation to the lungs; good for asthma; strong anticancer effect.

UME/SHO/BANCHA DRINK

Pour one cup of bancha twig tea over the meat of 1/2 -1 umeboshi plum and one teaspoon of tamari or soy sauce. Stir and drink hot.

Uses: strengthens the blood, regulates the digestion, stimulates circulation.

UMEBOSHI KUZU DRINK

Dissolve a heaping teaspoon of kuzu root powder into one cup of cold water. Add 1/2 of an umeboshi plum and a dash of soy sauce. Bring the mixture to a boil, reduce the heat to simmering, and stir constantly until the liquid becomes a transparent gelatin. A little bit of fresh grated ginger also can be added.

Uses: strengthens digestion, increases vitality, and can relieve general fatigue.

AME KUZU DRINK

Dissolve one heaping teaspoon of kuzu root powder into one cup of cold water. Add 1-2 teaspoons brown rice syrup or barley malt, or one-half cup apple juice. Bring to a boil over medium flame, stirring constantly, until the liquid becomes translucent. Drink while hot.

Uses: relaxes mind and body. It is especially recommended for children and can bring down fever in small children. It is also good for stomach and intestinal problems, hypoglycemia, premenstrual and menstrual cramps, and tension.

Acupoint Names

LUNG MERIDIAN

	Japanese	Chinese
LU 1	Chufu	Zhongfu
LU 2	Unmon	Yunmen
LU 3	Tenpu	Tianfu
LU 4	Kyohaku	Xiabai
LU 5	Shakutaku	Chize
LU 6	Kosai	Kongzui
LU 7	Rekketsu	Lieque
LU 8	Keikyo	Jingqu
LU 9	Taien	Taiyuan
LU 10	Gyosai	Yuji
LU 11	Shosho	Shaoshang

LARGE INTESTINE MERIDIAN

	Japanese	Chinese
LI 1	Shoyo	Shangyang
LI 2	Jikan	Erjian
LI 3	Sankan	Sanjian
LI 4	Gokoku	Hegu
LI 5	Yokei	Yangxi
LI 6	Henreki	Pianli
LI 7	Onryu	Wenliu
LI 8	Geren	Xianlian
LI 9	Joren	Shanglian
LI 10	Te-no-Sanri	Shousanli
LI 11	Kyokuchi	Quchi
LI 12	Churyo	Zhouliao
LI 13	Te-no-Gori	Hand-Wuli
LI 14	Hiju	Binao
LI 15	Kengu	Jianyu
LI 16	Kokotsu	Jugu
LI 17	Tentei	Tianding
LI 18	Futotsu	Neck-Futu
LI 19	Karyo	Nose-Heliao
LI 20	Geiko	Yingxiang

STOMACH MERIDIAN

	Japanese	Chinese		Japanese	Chinese
ST 1	Shokyu	Chengqi	ST 24	Katsunikumon	Huaroumen
ST 2	Shihaku	Sibai	ST 25	Tensu	Tianshu
ST 3	Koryo	Nose-Juliao	ST 26	Gairyo	Wailing
ST 4	Chiso	Dicang	ST 27	Daiko	Daju
ST 5	Daigei	Daying	ST 28	Suido	Shuidao
ST 6	Kyosha	Jiache	ST 29	Kirai	Guilai
ST 7	Gekan	Xiaguan	ST 30	Kisho	Qichong
ST 8	Zui	Touwei	ST 31	Hikan	Biguan
ST 9	Jingei	Renying	ST 32	Fukuto	Femur-Futu
ST 10	Suitotsu	Shuitu	ST 33	Inshi	Yinshi
ST 11	Kisha	Qishe	ST 34	Ryokyu	Liangqiu
ST 12	Ketsubon	Quepen	ST 35	Tokubi	Dubi
ST 13	Kiko	Qihu	ST 36	Ashi-no-Sanri	Zusanli
ST 14	Kobo	Kufang	ST 37	Jokokyu	Shangjuxu
ST 15	Okuei	Wuyi	ST 38	Joko	Tiaokou
ST 16	Yoso	Yingchuang	ST 39	Gekokyo	Xiajuxu
ST 17	Nyuchu	Ruzhong	ST 40	Horyu	Fenglong
ST 18	Nyukon	Rugen	ST 41	Kaikei	Jiexi
ST 19	Fuyo	Burong	ST 42	Shoyo	Chongyang
ST 20	Shoman	Chengman	ST 43	Kankoku	Xiangu
ST 21	Ryomon	Liangmen	ST 44	Naitei	Neiting
ST 22	Kanmon	Guanmen	ST 45	Reida	Lidui
ST 23	Tai-itsu	Taiyi			

SPLEEN MERIDIAN

	Japanese	Chinese		Japanese	Chinese
SP 1	Impaku	Yinbai	SP 12	Shomon	Chongmen
SP 2	Daito	Dadu	SP 13	Fusha	Fushe
SP 3	Taihaku	Taibai	SP 14	Fukketsu	Fujie
SP 4	Koson	Gongsun	SP 15	Daio	Daheng
SP 5	Shokyu	Shangqiu	SP 16	Fuku-ai	Fuai
SP 6	Saninko	Sanyinjiao	SP 17	Shokutoku	Shidou
SP 7	Rokoku	Lougu	SP 18	Tenkei	Tianxi
SP 8	Chiki	Diji	SP 19	Kyokyo	Xiongxiang
SP 9	Inryosen	Yinlingquan	SP 20	Shuei	Zhourong
SP 10	Kekkai	Xuehai	SP 21	Daiho	Dabao
SP 11	Kimon	Jimen			

HEART MERIDIAN

	Japanese	**Chinese**
HT 1	Kyokusen	Jiquan
HT 2	Seirei	Qingling
HT 3	Shokai	Shaohai
HT 4	Reido	Lingdao
HT 5	Tsuri	Tongli
HT 6	Ingeki	Yinxi
HT 7	Shinmon	Shenmen
HT 8	Shofu	Shaofu
HT 9	Shosho	Shaochong

SMALL INTESTINE MERIDIAN

	Japanese	**Chinese**
SI 1	Shotaku	Shaoze
SI 2	Zenkoku	Qiangu
SI 3	Gokei	Houxi
SI 4	Wankotsu	Hand-Wangu
SI 5	Yokoku	Yanggu
SI 6	Yoro	Yanglao
SI 7	Shisei	Zhizheng
SI 8	Shokai	Xiaohai
SI 9	Kentai	Jianzhen
SI 10	Juyu	Naoshu
SI 11	Tenso	Tianzong
SI 12	Heifu	Bingfeng
SI 13	Kyokuen	Quyuan
SI 14	Kengaiyu	Jianwaishu
SI 15	Kenchuyu	Jianzhongshu
SI 16	Tenso	Tianchuang
SI 17	Tenyo	Tianrong
SI 18	Kenryo	Quanliao
SI 19	Chokyu	Tinggong

BLADDER MERIDIAN

	Japanese	Chinese		Japanese	Chinese
BL 1	Seimei	Jingming	BL 35	Eyo	Huiyang
BL 2	Sanchiko	Zanzhu	BL 36	Shofu	Chengfu
BL 3	Bisho	Meichong	BL 37	Inmon	Yinmen
BL 4	Kyokusa	Quchai	BL 38	Fugeki	Fuxi
BL 5	Gosho	Wuchu	BL 39	Iyo	Weiyang
BL 6	Shoko	Chengguang	BL 40	Ichu	Weizhong
BL 7	Tsuten	Tongtian	BL 41	Fubun	Fufen
BL 8	Rakkyaku	Luoque	BL 42	Hakko	Pohu
BL 9	Gyokuhcin	Yuzhen	BL 43	Koko	Gaohuangshu
BL 10	Tenchu	Tianzhu	BL 44	Shindo	Shentang
BL 11	Daijo	Dashu	BL 45	Iki	Yixi
BL 12	Fumon	Fengmen	BL 46	Kakukan	Geguan
BL 13	Haiyu	Feishu	BL 47	Konmon	Hunmen
BL 14	Ketsuinyu	Jueyinshu	BL 48	Yoko	Yanggang
BL 15	Shinyu	Xinshu	BL 49	Isha	Yishi
BL 16	Tokuyu	Dushu	BL 50	Iso	Weicang
BL 17	Kakuyu	Geshu	BL 51	Komon	Huangmen
BL 18	Kanyu	Ganshu	BL 52	Shishitsu	Zhishi
BL 19	Tanyu	Danshu	BL 53	Koko	Baohuang
BL 20	Hiyu	Pishu	BL 54	Chippen	Zhibian
BL 21	Iyu	Weishu	BL 55	Goyo	Heyang
BL 22	Sanshoyu	Sanjiaoshu	BL 56	Shokin	Chengjin
BL 23	Jinyu	Shenshu	BL 57	Shozan	Chengshan
BL 24	Kikaiyu	Qihaishu	BL 58	Hiyo	Feiyang
BL 25	Daichoyu	Dachangshu	BL 59	Fuyo	Fuyang
BL 26	Kangenyu	Guanyuanshu	BL 60	Konron	Kunlun
BL 27	Shochoyu	Xiaochangshu	BL 61	Bokushin	Pushen
BL 28	Bokoyu	Pangguangshu	BL 62	Shinmyaku	Shenmai
BL 29	Churoyu	Zhonglushu	BL 63	Kinmon	Jinmen
BL 30	Hakkanyu	Baihuanshu	BL 64	Keikotsu	Jinggu
BL 31	Joryo	Shangliao	BL 65	Sokkotsu	Shugu
BL 32	Jiryo	Ciliao	BL 66	Ashi-no-Tsukoku	Foot-Tonggu
BL 33	Churyo	Zhongliao	BL 67	Shi-in	Zhiyin
BL 34	Geryo	Xialiao			

KIDNEY MERIDIAN

	Japanese	Chinese		Japanese	Chinese
KI 1	Yusen	Yongquan	KI 15	Chuchu	Abdomen-Zhongzhu
KI 2	Nenkoku	Rangu	KI 16	Koyu	Huangshu
KI 3	Taikei	Taixi	KI 17	Shokyoku	Shangqu
KI 4	Daisho	Dazhong	KI 18	Sekikan	Shiguan
KI 5	Suisen	Shuiquan	KI 19	Into	Yindu
KI 6	Shokai	Zhaohai	KI 20	Hara-no-Tsukoku	Abdomen-Tonggu
KI 7	Fukuryu	Fuliu	KI 21	Yumon	Youmen
KI 8	Koshin	Jiaoxin	KI 22	Horo	Bulang
KI 9	Chikuhin	Zhubin	KI 23	Shinpo	Shenfeng
KI 10	Inkoku	Yingu	KI 24	Reikyo	Lingxu
KI 11	Okotsu	Henggu	KI 25	Shinzo	Shencang
KI 12	Daikaku	Dahe	KI 26	Wakuchu	Yuzhong
KI 13	Kiketsu	Qixue	KI 27	Yufu	Shufu
KI 14	Shiman	Siman			

HEART GOVERNOR MERIDIAN

	Japanese	Chinese		Japanese	Chinese
HG 1	Tenchi	Tianchi	HG 5	Kanshi	Jianshi
HG 2	Tensen	Tianquan	HG 6	Naikan	Neiguan
HG 3	Kyokutaku	Quze	HG 7	Dairyo	Daling
HG 4	Gekimon	Ximen	HG 8	Rokyu	Laogong
			HG 9	Chusho	Zhongchong

TRIPLE HEATER (Sanjio) MERIDIAN

	Japanese	Chinese		Japanese	Chinese
TH 1	Kansho	Guanchong	TH 13	Jue	Naohui
TH 2	Ekimon	Yemen	TH 14	Kenryo	Jianliao
TH 3	Chusho	Hand-Zhongzhu	TH 15	Tenryo	Tianliao
TH 4	Yochi	Yangchi	TH 16	Tenyo	Tianyou
TH 5	Gaikan	Waiguan	TH 17	Eifu	Yifeng
TH 6	Shikko	Zhigou	TH 18	Keimyaku	Qimai
TH 7	Eso	Huizong	TH 19	Rosoku	Luxi
TH 8	Sanyoraku	Sanyangluo	TH 20	Kakuson	Jiaosun
TH 9	Shitoku	Sidu	TH 21	Jimon	Ermem
TH 10	Tensei	Tianjing	TH 22	Waryo	Ear-Heliao
TH 11	Seireien	Qinglengyuan	TH 23	Shichikuku	Sizhukong
TH 12	Shoreki	Xiaoluo			

GALL BLADDER MERIDIAN

	Japanese	Chinese		Japanese	Chinese
GB 1	Doshiryo	Tongziliao	GB 23	Chokin	Zhejin
GB 2	Choe	Tinghui	GB 24	Jitsugetsu	Riyue
GB 3	Kakushujin	Shangguan	GB 25	Keimon	Jingmen
GB 4	Ganen	Hanyan	GB 26	Taimyaku	Daimai
GB 5	Kenro	Xuanlu	GB 27	Gosu	Wushu
GB 6	Kenri	Zuanli	GB 28	Ido	Weidao
GB 7	Kyokubin	Qubin	GB 29	Kyoryo	Femur-Juliao
GB 8	Sokkoku	Shuaigu	GB 30	Kancho	Huantiao
GB 9	Tensho	Tianchong	GB 31	Fushi	Fengshi
GB 10	Fuhaku	Fubai	GB 32	Chutoku	Femur-Zhongdu
GB 11	Atama-no-Kyo-in	Head-Qiaoyin	GB 33	Ashi-no-Yokan	Xiyangguan
GB 12	Kankotsu	Head-Wangu	GB 34	Yoryosen	Yanglingquan
GB 13	Honshin	Benshen	GB 35	Yoko	Yangjiao
GB 14	Yohaku	Yangbai	GB 36	Gaikyu	Waiqiu
GB 15	Atama-no-Rinkyu	Head-Linqi	GB 37	Komei	Guangming
GB 16	Mikuso	Muchuang	GB 38	Yoho	Yangfu
GB 17	Shoei	Zhengying	GB 39	Kensho	Xuanzhong
GB 18	Shorei	Chengling	GB 40	Kyukyo	Qiuxu
GB 19	Noku	Naokong	GB 41	Ashi-no-Rinkyu	Foot-Linqi
GB 20	Fuchi	Fengchi	GB 42	Chigoe	Diwuhui
GB 21	Kensei	Jianjing	GB 43	Kyokei	Xiaxi
GB 22	Eneki	Yuanye	GB 44	Ashi-no-Kyo-in	Foot-Qiaoyin

LIVER MERIDIAN

	Japanese	Chinese		Japanese	Chinese
LV 1	Daiton	Dadun	LV 8	Kyokusen	Ququan
LV 2	Kokan	Xingjian	LV 9	Impo	Yinbao
LV 3	Taisho	Taichong	LV 10	Ashi-no-Gori	Femur-Wuli
LV 4	Chuho	Zhongfeng	LV 11	Inren	Yinlian
LV 5	Reiko	Ligou	LV 12	Kyumyaku	Jimai
LV 6	Chuto	Foot-Zhongdu	LV 13	Shomon	Zhangmen
LV 7	Shitsukan	Xiguan	LV 14	Kimon	Qimen

GOVERNING VESSEL MERIDIAN

	Japanese	Chinese		Japanese	Chinese
GV 1	Chokyu	Changqiang	GV15	Amon	Yamen
GV 2	Yoyu	Yaoshu	GV 16	Fufu	Fengfu
GV 3	Koshi-no-Yokan	Yaoyangguan	GV 17	Noko	Naohu
GV 4	Meimon	Mingmen	GV 18	Kyokan	Qiangjian
GV 5	Kensu	Xuanshu	GV 19	Gocho	Houding
GV 6	Sekichu	Jizhong	GV 20	Hyakue	Baihui
GV 7	Chusu	Zhongshu	GV 21	Zencho	Qianding
GV 8	Kinshuku	Jinsuo	GV 22	Shine	Xinhui
GV 9	Shiyo	Zhiyang	GV 23	Josei	Shangxing
GV 10	Reidai	Lingtai	GV 24	Shintei	Shenting
GV 11	Shindo	Shendao	GV 25	Soryo	Suliao
GV 12	Shinchu	Shenzhu	GV 26	Suiko	Renzhong
GV 13	Todo	Taodao	GV 27	Datnan	Duiduan
GV 14	Daitsui	Dazhui	GV 28	Ginko	Mouth-Yinjiao

CONCEPTION VESSEL MERIDIAN

	Japanese	Chinese		Japanese	Chinese
CV 1	Ein	Huiyin	CV 13	Jokan	Shangwan
CV 2	Kyokkotsu	Qugu	CV 14	Koketsu	Juque
CV 3	Chukyoku	Zhongji	CV 15	Kyubi	Jiuwei
CV 4	Kangenri	Guanyuan	CV 16	Chutei	Zhongting
CV 5	Sekimon	Shimen	CV 17	Danchu	Shangzhong
CV 6	Kikai	Qihai	CV 18	Gyokudo	Yutang
CV 7	Inko	Abdomen-Yinjiao	CV 19	Shikyu	Chest-Zigong
CV 8	Shiketsu	Shenque	CV 20	Kagai	Huagai
CV 9	Shibun	Shuifen	CV 21	Senki	Xuanji
CV 10	Gekan	Xiawan	CV 22	Tentotsu	Tiantu
CV 11	Kenri	Jianli	CV 23	Rensen	Lianquan
CV 12	Chukan	Zhongwan	CV 24	Shosho	Chengjian

About the Authors

SHIZUKO YAMAMOTO is recognized as one of the world's leading shiatsu practitioners and macrobiotic consultants and the creator of the Macrobiotic Shiatsu style. She has led seminars in the United States, Europe, and Japan for over 40 years. She has dedicated herself to spreading the simple message— "live according to nature." To further worldwide communication in the natural healing field, she initiated the International Macrobiotic Shiatsu Society. She has authored several books including *Barefoot Shiatsu*, *The Shiatsu Handbook*, and *Whole Health Shiatsu*. Her books have been translated into seven languages. She is a certified instructor in the American Organization for Bodywork Therapies of Asia (AOBTA) and the National Commission for the Certification of Acupuncture and Oriental Medicine (NCCAOM).

PATRICK McCARTY is the former director of a natural health education organization in northern California. He studied at the Shanghai College of Traditional Chinese Medicine. He has co-written five books and is editor of "Healthways", the newsletter of the International Macrobiotic Shiatsu Society. Ms. Yamamoto and Mr. McCarty's books are now part of the Smithsonian Institute's Complementary Health collection. He has consulted with government officials in the U.S. and Cuba regarding macrobiotics and shiatsu. He is a certified instructor (C.I.) in AOBTA and National Board Certified in Asian Bodywork Therapy (NCCAOM). He is also approved by the National Certification Board for Therapeutic Massage and Bodywork (NCBTMB) as a continuing education Approved Provider.

International Macrobiotic Shiatsu Society is a membership organization open to everyone. Members receive the I.M.S.S. newsletter *"Healthways"* from time to time. Annual membership fee is $25 in U.S. ($30 foreign). Send check to: I.M.S.S., Attention: Membership, 2807 Wright Avenue, Winter Park, FL 32789.

> Other **Books Available**
>
> *20-Minute Shiatsu* by Yamamoto & McCarty
>
> *Beginners Guide to Shiatsu* by Patrick McCarty
>
> **Media Available**
>
> *Barefoot Shiatsu* (on DVD)
>
> *Macrobiotic Shiatsu Workbook* (CD, Acrobat pdf file-text viewed on computer)

For more information visit our web site at: **imss.macrobiotic.net**

Notes